Developed by:
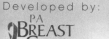
PA
BREAST
CANCER
COALITION

BREAST CANCER:
Covered or Not?

A guide on insurance

Dr. Linda M. Rhodes
and Pat Halpin-Murphy

Published in the United States of America by

Pascoe Publishing, Inc.

Rocklin, California

www.pascoepublishing.com

ISBN: 1-929862-53-9

05   06   07   08   10   9   8   7   6   5   4   3   2   1

Printed in the United States of America

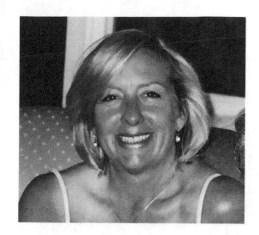

To Carey Lackman Slease

DEDICATION

The Pennsylvania Breast Cancer Coalition dedicates this insurance guidebook to Carey Lackman Slease, a truly inspiring and powerful woman. Carey was chief of staff to U.S. Senator, Arlen Specter, and lost her battle with breast cancer in July of 2004. She was one of the first women to serve as chief of staff in the U.S. Senate, and was acclaimed as one of Pennsylvania's most politically powerful women.

"Carey was very accomplished, brilliant, energetic and passionate. She made a difference in the lives of all who knew her, and her passing leaves a void that can't be filled."

—United States Senator Arlen Specter

Acknowledgements

We've dreamt for quite a long time of developing an insurance guide to empower women coping with breast cancer and because of the following individuals and organizations, this dream is now a reality. We'd like to give a special thanks to: Senator Arlen Specter for shepherding funding our way and remaining our steadfast advocate, our former Governor Tom Ridge and Michele Ridge (who chaired the Pennsylvania Breast Cancer Coalition as First Lady) for their gift toward publishing this guide and Nazareth Hospital of Philadelphia for their gift toward printing.

We are also very grateful for the pro-bono services of Pavone Advertising whose very talented designers created our beautiful cover and graphics design of the guide.

We're indebted to our Expert Panel who spent a day advising us on the insurance issues facing women with breast cancer: Sharlene Bence, RN, Andrews & Patel Associates, PC; Cheryl Delsite, breast cancer survivor; G. June Hoch, PBCC Board member; Haya Jacqui Howells, RN, Sacred Heart Hospital; Yen Lucas, PA Insurance Department; Gayle Mills, Office of Senator Arlen Specter; Diane Koken, PA Insurance Commissioner; Helen Norton, Office of Minority Leader H. William DeWeese, PA House of Representatives; Brent O'Connell, MD, Medical Director, Highmark Blue Shield and PBCC Board member; Bradley Shopp, Triad Strategies; Jennifer Raviv, PhRMA; Helen Willis, RN, Sacred Heart Hospital; Susan Zeigler, Holy Spirit Health System; Kathleen Zitka, PA Department of Health.

Three individuals stand out among our PBCC staff for their excellent management of the project and thorough fact-finding: Heather Hibshman, Executive Director, Dolores Magro, Director of Development & Patient Advocate, and Tricia Grove, Administrative Director.

Insurance and benefit issues are complicated and we'd like to thank our technical reviewers who helped us with accuracy: Yen Lucas, PA Insurance Department; the team at Highmark Blue Shield under the leadership of Brent O'Connell, MD; Connie Bires, PA Department of Public Welfare; Celene Funk, PA Department of Health; Jack Vogelsong, APPRISE Coordinator, PA Department of Aging; and Tom Snedden, Director of PACE/PACENET.

And finally, thanks to the sage editing eye of Peg Albert of Matrix Communications Associates, who made sure you would understand what we're saying.

This project was funded by a grant from the Centers for Disease Control.

About the Authors

Dr. Linda Rhodes is former Secretary of Aging for the state of Pennsylvania who oversaw two billion dollars worth of long term care services. She created the award-winning Family Caregiving Program, helping thousands of families care for their loved ones at home. She now consults nationally for state governments on health care and education policy and performance.

Rhodes is an accomplished author and recently won two *2005 National Mature Media Awards* for her book, *Should Mom be left alone? Should Dad be driving?* (New American Library 2005) and her popular weekly newspaper column, *Our Parents, Ourselves.* Her book, *Caregiving as Your Parents Age* (Penguin Group USA 2005), receives excellent reviews from consumers and professionals alike. She has also conducted research studies in long term care and public health.

Dr. Rhodes has appeared on national talk shows such as *CNBC* and *Living it up with Ali and Jack.* She's been quoted in the *Wall Street Journal, More Magazine, Better Homes & Garden, Family Circle* and, *The New York Times,* along with numerous other newspapers and magazines. She is frequently interviewed for radio shows nationwide.

Rhodes holds a doctorate from Teachers College, Columbia University and is a popular speaker at conferences on aging and health care throughout the country. She found her inspiration to write this book from her admiration of her mother-in-law, Bernice L. Schnurer, who recently died of breast cancer amidst a brave and courageous fight. You can learn more about Linda Rhodes at www.lindarhodes.com.

Pat Halpin-Murphy is the President and Founder of the Pennsylvania Breast Cancer Coalition. Founded in June of 1993, the PBCC is organized statewide through a regional and county system designed to extend public awareness of breast cancer, and to encourage increased public and private funding for research, legislative advocacy and high quality screening, diagnosis and treatment.

Pat grew up in Philadelphia, earning a Master of Science degree in Economics from Drexel University, a Master of Arts degree in Political Science from the University of Pennsylvania and a Bachelor of Science degree in Education from West Chester University.

She is a Gubernatorial Appointee to the Pennsylvania Cancer Advisory Board and chairs the Income Tax Check-Off for Breast and Cervical Cancer Research Committee, which has designated over $1.5 million in grants to outstanding researchers across the state. Pat acts as an Advocate Member, representing breast cancer survivors, on the Board of Directors for the NSABP (National Surgical Adjuvant Breast and Bowel Project). In addition to her role as an Advocate Member, Pat chairs the NSABP Patient Advisory Board, which reviews new proposals and protocols for clinical trials. She also serves as a member of the University of Pennsylvania Breast Cancer Advocacy Board for the P2 trial. Additionally, Pat serves on the Patient Advocacy Committee of the Coalition of National Cancer Cooperative Groups, Inc. and on the corporate board for Highmark Blue Shield.

Pat has received numerous awards for her commitment to public service, including the "Distinguished Service to State Government" award, presented by the National Governors' Association; the "Women Change America" award, presented by the PA Commission for Women; and the "Infinity Award," presented by Villanova University.

Pat is an avid political scholar, committed public servant and outspoken advocate living in Ambler, Pennsylvania.

Contents

INTRODUCTION

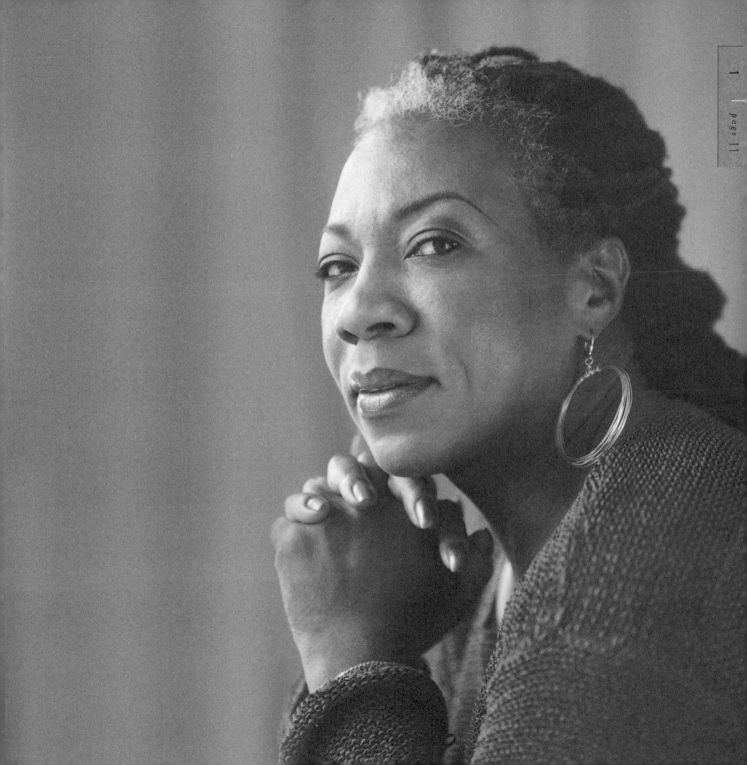

How to use this guide

We talked to hundreds of women in developing this guide to better understand their insurance experiences while they sought breast cancer treatment. We also gained insights from health care professionals who interact with insurance companies on behalf of their patients. As a result, we developed a guide that touches upon the most frequent insurance-related questions, issues and concerns that women encounter while they pursue treatment for breast cancer.

We organized the guide according to various circumstances: Part II offers information on a wide range of topics that apply to everyone; Part III guides you down the "insurance path" that relate to your unique situation; and Part IV prepares you for appealing denials and being on guard for potential hospital billing mistakes. Part V offers a "Tool Kit" providing you with a glossary of insurance terms, a resource list, a master check list of questions you should ask your insurance company and sample letters to request family medical leave,

DISCLAIMER

This guide is intended to help you understand your protections under federal and state law. The authors have made every attempt to assure that the information presented in this guide is accurate as of the date of publication. Our guide, however, is an overview and should not be used as a substitute for legal, accounting, or other expert professional advice. Readers should consult insurance regulators or other competent professionals for guidance in making health insurance decisions. The authors, publisher, and the Pennsylvania Breast Cancer Coalition specifically disclaim any personal liability, loss or risk incurred as a consequence of the use and application, either directly or indirectly, of any information presented in this guide.

This publication was supported by Grant Number H75/CCH324099-01 from the Centers for Disease Control. Its contents are solely the responsibility of the authors and do not necessarily represent the official views of CDC.

reasonable accommodations to maintain your job and additional clarification from your insurer when your physician's request for a medically necessary procedure or surgery has been denied.

Our mission is to help you navigate the insurance maze by acting as your personal guide and compass. We know that your first goal is to gain back your health and we want you to focus all of your energy on that goal. Perhaps you have a family member or trusted friend who can use this guide on your behalf to tackle insurance issues while you focus on your treatment. Best wishes in your recovery. We hope that — on the insurance side of things — we've made life a little bit easier for you and your loved ones.

INFORMATION
for everyone

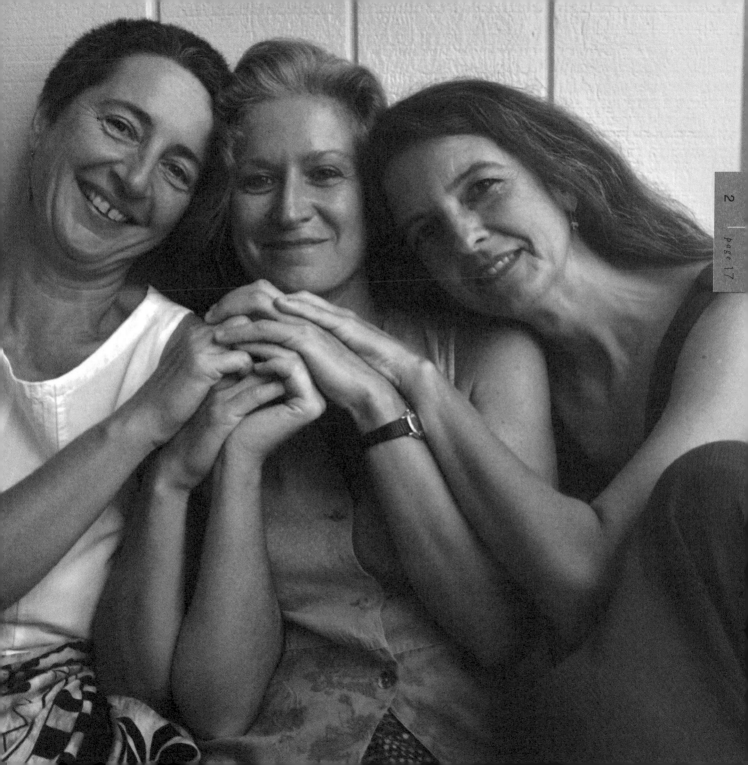

1. WHERE TO TURN FOR HELP
with insurance claims

Most women will tell you that despite the guiding hand they receive from professionals on how to navigate the breast cancer insurance maze, they still need their own compass to make sure that their insurers pay for their care. Grab a nice portfolio with folders to start keeping track of your insurance papers. You might want to consider creating folders that follow the subject outline of this book. Our intent is to act as your compass — directing you toward successful coverage for your care amid the twists and turns along your treatment journey.

There are three basic "guides" that can scout the lay of the land for you regarding third party coverage for your treatment and care. They are:

Your doctor's office

By now you've met your oncologist, who should be directing and coordinating your care. Ask the nurse manager of the office whom you should talk to about insurance coverage. Some doctor's offices employ an insurance coordinator who will help you, while others may offer the services of a social worker. Whoever this person is, introduce yourself and ask what procedures you should follow to request advice when and if you need it. This individual has access to the latest data and software regarding insurance coverage, laws, and regulations governing third party reimbursement. Don't be shy about asking for assistance.

The cancer center

If you receive care at a cancer center, there will be insurance coordinators and/or social workers who will meet with you to go over your insurance coverage as it relates to the treatment and care you'll receive at the cancer center. Social workers also provide information on possible benefits that you may be eligible for, such as a pharmaceutical program or disability benefits from Social Security, and how to apply. They'll also know of a wide variety of services and programs ranging from home health services, day care, credit and budget assistance, therapy, self-help groups, transportation, legal assistance and free medical clinics, to hospice care that may assist you. You may need to ask for an appointment with the social worker, if one isn't automatically assigned to you. The appointment will be well worth your time. Hospitals also employ social workers, so feel free to ask for their assistance during a hospital stay.

Your employer

If you are working, your employer is a key player on your "cancer care team." Even though he or she isn't providing direct medical care, your employer in many ways acts as the gateway for access to your care and can advise you on the finances of your treatment in terms of what your policy will cover and the workplace accommodations that may help you juggle your care and your job. Ask to speak to the human resource representative or the employee benefits manager. This should be one of your first appointments.

2. THREE QUESTIONS
you'll always want to ask

1. Is your employer self-insured or insured by a third party carrier?

If you are employed, ask your benefits manager whether the company or organization you work for is *self-insured* or *buys* its insurance from a third party. Depending on that answer, state and federal laws about breast cancer coverage may apply differently. When you know the answer, go to Part III (Path 1) of this book to learn what this means for you.

2. Am I covered?

Before you begin any major treatment or make any significant purchase (e.g., prosthesis), always ask: *Is this covered under my policy?* Whoever prescribes your treatment should be able to answer this question. If not, check with your insurer before you proceed. This applies to Medicare beneficiaries as well as those with private insurance. Never assume that just because the doctor is prescribing it, your treatment is covered.

3. How much do I have to pay?

If you are forced to pay for treatment, supplies, medications or a device, ask how much this will cost and whether there are any programs that might help defray these costs. Go to the Resources Section of our "Tool Kit" in Part V to find a list of resources that are available for you.

3. Do you qualify for Social Security Disability Income?

If you've ever worked, you know what it's like to see those Social Security withdrawals from your paycheck. Most of us know that some of this money is being stowed away for our retirement, but it also contributes toward disability benefits if you should ever become so disabled that you're no longer able to work. That's the good news. Proving that you are no longer able to work isn't easy, however, and the definition of being disabled is very narrow.

Here are the basics on Social Security Disability Income (SSDI) benefits:

- Social Security pays only for TOTAL disability. You are considered disabled if you cannot do the work that you performed before your breast cancer and you cannot adjust to other work because of your medical condition(s). In other words, the disability must be severe.

- You must have worked long enough—and recently enough—to qualify for disability benefits. Social Security calculates your work credits based upon your total yearly wages or self-employment income. You can earn up to four credits each year. Generally, you need 40 credits, half of which were earned in the last 10 years ending with the year you became disabled. However, younger workers may qualify with fewer credits.

- Your disability must also last or be expected to last for at least one year or to result in death.

TIP

You should apply for benefits as soon as you're disabled because it takes Social Security from three to six months to render a decision. If you are approved, your benefits do not begin until the sixth month of full disability.

There are three ways to apply for SSDI:

1. Go online to www.ssa.gov and complete your application online. You will find step-by-step guidelines on how to apply and answers to frequently asked questions regarding eligibility.

2. Call the toll-free Social Security telephone number at 1-800-772-1213. If you are deaf or hard of hearing, call them at TTY 1-800-325-0778.

3. Call or visit your local Social Security office, listed in the government pages of your phone book.

Even if you are turned down, it's smart to apply again. Some women have found that they were approved after they filed an appeal and their cases were reviewed a second time.

4. THE INSURANCE WORLD:
Two ways to look at it

Fee-for-service or managed care?

The insurance world changes daily and the lines that separate different types of plans from one another become increasingly blurred. But from a bird's eye view, two basic kinds of insurance plans emerge — those that allow their members to find their own healthcare providers and pay the provider a given fee for that service (fee-for-service), and those that manage the care for their members by directing care to a specified network of providers with whom they have negotiated reimbursement.

Fee-for-service: premiums, coinsurance, deductibles, and lifetime limits

In this instance, the medical provider (usually a physician or hospital) is paid a fee for each service that is rendered to you as a patient. In fee-for-service plans, you see the doctor of your choice and you, your doctor, or the hospital submits a claim to your insurance company for reimbursement. Covered medical expenses eligible for

TIP ✎

Always ask your medical provider whether your insurer's payment will be accepted as payment in full. If it is not, then you're going to have to pick up the difference. For example, let's say your doctor charges $120 for a service but the reasonable and customary fee for that service is $100; your insurer will likely pay $80 towards the bill and you will pay your $20 coinsurance PLUS you'll pay the additional $20 that your doctor is charging over the "reasonable and customary fee" set by your insurance plan. If this will become a great expense to you, it might be smart to find another medical provider who will accept what your insurer will pay as payment in full.

Medicare providers do accept what Medicare assigns as payment in full.

reimbursement are listed in the benefits summary of your insurance plan. You will likely be reimbursed for some, but generally not all, of the cost of the service provided to you. How much you receive depends upon the provisions of the policy on coinsurance and deductibles.

Fee-for-service. These plans, whether private or government-sponsored such as traditional or original Medicare, expect you to pay some of the costs of your health care. How much the insurer pays for your health care and how much you pay depends upon the plan that you've joined. But this, in general, is how it works:

Premiums. Quite simply, this is the amount you pay monthly, quarterly, or annually to be a member of a health plan that, in return, agrees to pay varying amounts toward your healthcare expenses.

Coinsurance. The portion that you pay toward a medical expense covered by your plan is called coinsurance. Many policies that are based upon paying a fee for each service you receive by a medical provider (fee-for-service plans) reimburse your doctor bills at 80 percent of the "reasonable and customary charge" for medical services. This charge is based upon the prevailing costs of offering these services in the geographic area from which you are receiving this service.

You pay the remaining 20 percent of the bill, which is, in other words, your coinsurance.

Many fee-for-service plans pay hospital expenses in full while others reimburse at the common 80/20 level described above. Whenever possible, check with your plan first, before embarking upon a major medical expense.

Deductibles. Under most plans, you will pay a set amount of your medical expenses every year before your insurer will begin paying its share. This amount usually runs into the hundreds of dollars. Let's say your deductible is $300 per year and the beginning of your policy's annual cycle is January. That means you will be paying out the first $300 of your medical expenses in full. Only after you have reached this threshold (your deductible) will your insurance plan start picking up its share (usually 80 percent), and you'll be back to paying your 20 percent coinsurance.

You will usually find that your premium payments will be lower if you agree to pay a higher deductible each year.

Out-of-pocket maximum. Once your expenses reach a certain amount in a given calendar year, many insurers will start paying your full bill based upon the reasonable and customary fee for your covered benefits. Your doctor, however, may still bill you above what the insurer pays. This maximum is often thousands of dollars, but it protects you from catastrophic expenses.

Lifetime limits. Policies usually set a limit on the amount they will pay toward your medical expenses throughout your life. Once you've exhausted that amount, you pay for everything in full. Given the rising costs of medical care and the fact that we're living longer, most experts recommend that you find a policy with a lifetime limit of at least $1 million.

Managed Care: HMO, PPO, POS and the list goes on

Managed care plans essentially do what their name implies: they generally *manage* your care by paying providers who join their network a negotiated amount to provide care to you. These "managed plans" usually provide comprehensive health services and offer financial incentives for you to use healthcare providers who belong to the plan. Your insurer has negotiated cost-saving rates with these providers.

These plans are referred to as "managed care," and they come in three major types:

Health Maintenance Organizations (HMO)

If you join an HMO, you'll pay a monthly or quarterly premium and a modest copayment for office visits and for every prescription. Most members find they pay relatively few out-of-pocket expenses for medical care compared to people who use the fee-for-service system. You must, however, use the doctors and hospitals that participate in or are part of the HMO. Your expense usually consists of copayments and, of course, your premiums to join the HMO. Most HMO members do not pay deductibles or coinsurance.

In an HMO you will choose a Primary Care Physician (PCP) who will coordinate your care and will refer you to specialists, who are also "participating providers" in the HMO network. In special circumstances, patients enrolled in an HMO may be referred to providers outside the HMO network and still receive coverage. However, this must be approved *first*. HMOs provide direct care to their patients, and in many cases, you'll go to one of their medical facilities to receive your care.

Some HMOs have contractual arrangements with Individual Practice Associations (IPA). In this instance, the IPA negotiates fees with independent physicians who work in their own private practices and see both fee-for-service patients and HMO enrollees.

Preferred Provider Organizations (PPO)

Like HMOs, these organizations have contracts with a network of doctors, hospitals, and other providers to secure better rates for your care. However, unlike the HMO, a PPO may allow you to go out of the network to receive care. As a result, these plans usually charge a higher coinsurance when you see physicians outside of the network, and you may find premiums for PPOs to be higher than a HMO.

Point of Service Plans (POS)

These plans also offer a network of doctors, hospitals, and other providers who have agreed to accept reduced rates for healthcare services, which, in turn, makes the premiums you pay more reasonable than in a traditional fee-for-service plan. Generally these plans operate similarly to the PPOs, however, they might require you to work with a Primary Care Physician to coordinate your care.

5. IN-NETWORK AND OUT-OF-NETWORK:
A world of difference

In most health plans, there are two levels of coverage: In-Network and Out-of-Network. Managed care plans have negotiated price breaks for their enrollees with a "network" of physicians, specialists, hospitals, and other healthcare providers. As a result, using network providers means less out of pocket expenses for you in the form of lower copayments, deductibles and coinsurance than if you use providers outside of your plan's network.

Out-of-Network physicians, specialists or other providers are not members of your plan's network and this means you will be responsible for amounts they charge that are in excess of your plan's "covered charges." Covered charges are usual, customary, and reasonable charges for a particular service or procedure predetermined by your plan. If you are enrolled in a managed care plan, there are rules you must follow to receive care from anyone outside of their network. Be sure to read your *Summary Plan Description* to learn what steps you need to take to see a specialist outside of the network.

In certain circumstances, your plan may allow you to see a provider who is not a member of your network. For example, you may require highly specialized medical care that is not available in your network or you may need to use Out-of-Network services in emergencies or when you are traveling. In emergency cases, let your plan know as soon as reasonably possible that you've received care outside of the network. You will need to work with your Primary Care Physician to arrange for highly specialized care that is not available in your plan's network.

If your health plan is a PPO (preferred provider organization) or a POS (point of service) plan that covers services provided by doctors or hospitals that are not part of the plan's network, then be aware that if the Out-of-Network provider charges more than what the health plan claims is reasonable, you will likely pay the difference, plus any coinsurance.

TIP

If you are in a managed care plan, always check with your primary care physician (PCP) first before you see anyone outside of the network. In some instances, you might require a very specialized procedure that no one in the network can offer. The primary care physician can work with the plan to make arrangements for you to see someone outside of the network and to have it covered by the HMO.

6. PRE-EXISTING CONDITIONS and HIPAA

Probably one of your greatest worries is whether your breast cancer will be considered a pre-existing condition if you should lose your job and need to find health insurance. The Health Insurance Portability and Accountability Act (HIPAA) is a relatively new law that assures continued health insurance coverage for employees and their dependents. Insurers can impose only one 12-month waiting period for any pre-existing condition treated or diagnosed in the previous six months. If you have maintained continuous coverage without a break of more than 62 days, then your prior health insurance coverage will be credited toward the "pre-existing condition exclusion" period of your new insurer.

According to the U.S. Department of Labor, here are some other protections that the HIPAA law grants you:

- You cannot be denied eligibility for benefits or charged a higher premium based upon health factors of: health status, medical conditions either physical or mental, previous high claims use, genetic information, or disability.

- A group health plan or group health insurance issuer may not require you to pass a physical examination for enrollment.

- Time periods for pre-existing condition exclusions must be applied uniformly to all similarly situated individuals in the group's health plan. You cannot be treated differently because of your breast cancer.

- Group health plans may exclude coverage for a specific disease, limit or exclude benefits for certain types of treatments or drugs, or limit or exclude benefits based on a determination of whether the benefits are experimental or medically necessary *if the benefit restriction is applied uniformly to all similarly situated individuals* and is not directed at any individual participants or beneficiaries based on a health factor.

- A group health plan may not restrict your eligibility, benefits, or the effective date of coverage based on your confinement in a hospital or other healthcare facility.

In Pennsylvania, if you are HIPAA eligible, you are guaranteed the right to buy individual health insurance policies and are exempted from pre-existing condition exclusion periods. Blue Cross and Blue Shield plans operating in your region must offer you a choice of at least two state-approved policies. According to Georgetown University Health Policy Institute's *Consumer's Guide on Health Insurance,* you are HIPAA eligible if you meet all of the following criteria:

- You must have had 18 months of continuous creditable coverage, *at least the last day of which was under a group health plan*.

- You also must have used up any COBRA or state continuation coverage for which you were eligible. (See Part III, Path 1)

- You must not be eligible for Medicare, Medicaid, or a group health plan.

- You must not have health insurance. (If you know your group coverage is about to end, you can apply for coverage for which you *will* be HIPAA eligible.)

- You must apply for health insurance for which you are HIPAA eligible within 63 days of losing your prior coverage.

- Federal eligibility ends when you enroll in individual coverage, because the last day of your continuous health coverage must have been in a *group* plan. You can become HIPAA eligible again by maintaining continuous coverage and rejoining a group health plan.

If you have a question regarding your rights under HIPAA, contact the Employee Benefits Security Administration (EBSA) at 1-866-444-3272. You can also call or write to their regional Pennsylvania Office at:

> EBSA Philadelphia Regional Office
> Curtis Center
> 70 S. Independence Mall West
> Suite 870 West
> Philadelphia, PA 19106-3317
> Telephone: 1-215-861-5300

Or visit the Department of Labor website at www.dol.gov and enter the keyword HIPAA at the search function.

7. Clinical trials:
What are they and who pays?

What are they? Clinical trials are research studies that determine whether vaccines, drugs, new therapies, or new treatments are safe and effective. These trials are offered to humans after researchers have tested the various procedures in laboratories and on animals. An Institutional Review Board (IRB) must approve all clinical trials. This board consists of researchers, physicians, and consumers who review the proposed study and assure that it is safe and ethical and that the rights of those being studied are protected. Be aware, however, that the sponsoring institution of the study forms the IRB.

Besides receiving the go-ahead from an IRB, pharmaceutical companies must gain approval from the Food & Drug Administration (FDA), assuring that the animal and laboratory studies of the drug company were successful enough to warrant safe testing of humans.

There are usually four phases to clinical trials, with each phase expanding to test more people. For instance, a Phase I study will research a small group of 20 to 80 people; by Phase III, up to 3,000 people may be involved.

Frequently, patients in clinical trials are assigned either to a "study" group that receives the new treatment or to a "control" group that receives standard treatment or a placebo (an inactive pill, liquid, or powder with no treatment value, such as a sugar pill). It is unethical, however, to give a sick patient a placebo when there is a known beneficial treatment available.

TIP ✍

The "protocol" of a clinical trial is the plan of study for the research project; it describes the types of people who will be tested, the schedule of tests, treatment, medications, dosages, and length of time in the study.

The major benefit of participating in a clinical trial is to gain access to the latest "discovery" and, hopefully, the most advanced form of treatment.

TIP ✒

Be sure to consult your oncologist if you consider entering a clinical trial, as you will want your doctor to work with the clinical trial team. Ask for your doctor's opinion on the risks and benefits as they relate to your particular diagnosis. Remember: you can stop participating in the clinical trial at any time. This is absolutely voluntary.

Doing your research

Participating in a clinical trial can involve both benefits and risks so you'll want to do your homework to decide whether the benefits outweigh the risks. Your first step is to visit the National Institutes of Health (NIH) website at www.clinicaltrials.gov or call 1-800-411-1222. At the website you can simply search by topic: just enter the key words *breast cancer* and you'll immediately find clinical trials being conducted throughout the country, along with their contact information. You can also go to other links for further research on medical conditions and news on clinical trials from disease-related associations (e.g., American Cancer Society).

If you're wondering what you should be asking the doctors who run the clinical trial, NIH and other experts suggest that you ask:

- Who is sponsoring this study and who is funding this trial?

- Do you or the director have a financial stake in this treatment or drug?

- What can you show me to verify the credibility of the group sponsoring this clinical trial?

- What is the purpose of the study?

- How will my safety be monitored?

- Who is going to be in the study?

- Why do researchers believe the new treatment being tested may be effective? Has it been tested before? On how many people?

- What kinds of tests and treatments are involved?

- How do the possible risks, side effects, and benefits in the study compare with my current treatment?

- How might this trial affect my daily life?

- How long will the trial last?

- Will hospitalization be required?

- Who will pay for the treatment?

- Will I be reimbursed for other expenses? (e.g., travel and lodging)

- What type of long-term follow-up care is part of this study?

- How will I know that the treatment is working? Will results of the trials be provided to me?

- Who will be in charge of my care? How can I reach this person if I have complications?

Always take a family member or friend to the preliminary visit, bring a tape recorder, and carefully read the Informed Consent Form. This form should answer many of the questions listed above and clearly spell out the risks.

TIP

Before you participate in any clinical trial, secure in writing from your health plan an assurance that the usual and extra costs of patient care associated with the clinical trial will be covered. Make sure the sponsors of the clinical trial clearly spell out to you any costs not covered by your health plan or their clinic that will be your responsibility.

Clinical trials can be literal lifesavers. Just make sure that whoever offers the clinical trial is credible, is part of a highly regarded medical and/or academic institution, and is forthright about the risks and the funding source of the research study.

Who pays? According to the National Cancer Institute, costs related to clinical trials are identified as either patient care costs or research costs directly related to operating the study.

Patient care costs are divided into two basic categories:

1. Usual costs of care: these include such costs as doctor visits, hospital stays, clinical laboratory tests, and/or x-rays that occur whether you are participating in a trial or receiving standard treatment for your breast cancer. These costs are usually covered by a third-party health plan, such as Medicare or private insurance.

2. Extra costs of care: these include such costs as additional tests that may or may not be fully covered by the clinical trial sponsor and/or research institution. These costs are usually viewed as outside of the standard scope of treatment and care.

Research costs are those associated with conducting the trial, such as data collection and management, time spent by researcher physicians and nurses, analysis of results, and tests performed purely for research purposes. These costs are usually covered by the sponsoring organization, such as the National Cancer Institute (NCI) or a pharmaceutical company. These costs are *not* picked up by the patient.

How insurance companies decide what costs they'll cover

One of the determinants to whether or not a clinical trial is covered by insurance is whether your health plan considers the treatment you'll receive to be either *established* or *investigational*. Health plans usually determine the care and treatment as *established* if there is enough scientific data to prove that it is safe and effective. If the health plan does not find sufficient proof, the treatment may be deemed *investigational*.

If your health plan labels the clinical trial as *investigative* or *experimental*, payment for costs of patient care directly related to participating in the trial could very well be denied.

Health plans often spell out specific criteria that a trial must meet before they'll extend your coverage to pay for clinical trial costs. Here are some examples:

Sponsorship. The clinical trial must be sponsored by organizations whose review and oversight of the trial is scientifically rigorous and accredited.

TIP

Give your health plan a deadline by asking the hospital or cancer center to set a target date for the therapy. This will help to ensure that coverage decisions are made promptly.

Trial phase and type. Patient care costs are covered for clinical trials that the plan judges to be "medically necessary" on a case-by-case basis. Some plans will only cover clinical trials that are in the third phase of development, which means they have already been successful with greater numbers of people. The plan may require some proof of effectiveness before covering a Phase I or Phase II trial, which involves much smaller samples of people who have taken the trial's drug and/or treatment.

Cost neutrality. Coverage is limited to those clinical trials whose treatment costs aren't considered any more expensive than receiving the standard course of treatment. In other words, it is "cost neutral."

Lack of standard therapy. If no other standard of care or treatment is available for your condition, some plans will cover it.

Facility and qualifications. The facility and medical staff conducting the clinical trial must meet certain criteria by the health plan, especially when it comes to intensive forms of therapy (for example, high-dose chemotherapy with bone marrow or stem cell transplantation.)

How to increase your chance of coverage for a clinical trial

First, know the costs associated with the clinical trial. Ask your doctor or the trial's contact person about the costs that must be covered by you or your health plan. Get the details by asking:

- Are these costs significantly higher than those incurred by standard therapy?

- Have other patients in this trial been covered by their health plans?

- Have there been any persistent problems with plans covering this clinical trial?

- What's the track record of the trial's administrators in getting plans to cover patient care costs?

Second, know your health plan. This means reading your policy and carefully looking over the contract language. Perhaps a close friend or a family member can research this if you're too overwhelmed with all the healthcare decisions you're making. Look for any exclusion for "experimental or investigational treatment" and read it very closely to determine how the policy defines such treatment and under what conditions it will be covered. If it is not clearly defined, call the customer service phone number for your plan and get clarification in writing.

Work closely with your doctor: Talk with your physician about the paperwork he or she will submit to your health plan. If there have been problems with coverage in the past, you might ask your doctor or the hospital to send an information package to the plan that includes studies supporting the procedure's safety, benefits, and medical appropriateness.

Your information package might include:

- Publications from physician-reviewed literature about the proposed therapy that demonstrate patient benefits;

- A letter that uses the insurance contract's own language to explain why the treatment, screening method, or preventive measure should be covered;

- Letters from researchers that explain the clinical trial;

- Support letters from patient advocacy groups.

Be sure to keep for future reference your own copy of any materials that the doctor sends to your health plan. You'll also want to work closely with your company's benefits manager. This person may be helpful in enlisting the support of your employer to request coverage by the health plan.

8. LIMITS AND COVERAGE
for breast cancer procedures

Mammogram

What is it? A mammogram is a low-dose x-ray examination of the breast used to detect and diagnose breast disease in women, who may or may not have breast disease symptoms (e.g. lump, pain or nipple discharge). Mammography x-rays do not penetrate tissue as easily as the x-ray used for routine chest films. In order to allow for a lower dose x-ray, the breast is squeezed between 2 plates to spread the tissue apart. *Screening* mammograms are used to detect possible abnormalities of the breast for women who have no symptoms or signs of breast cancer. For many women, this is an annual exam to make sure they detect any possible signs of breast cancer at its earliest stages. *Diagnostic* mammograms provide a more detailed set of x-rays and are used to capture a more in-depth look at an abnormality (e.g. lump or nipple discharge).

Mammogram findings are reported by a standardized system known as Breast Imaging Reporting and Data System (BIRADS) ranging from Category 0 to Category 5; the higher the number of the category, the more suspicious the findings of the x-ray. A mammogram is not capable of determining that an area seen on the x-ray film is definitely cancer. If an area is suspicious then a sample of cells or tissue (biopsy) will need to be studied under a microscope. If you have had breast conserving surgery (e.g. lumpectomy) you will still need to continue having mammograms of both breasts.
The Mammography Quality Standards Act requires that clinics mail you an easy-to-understand report of your mammogram results within 30 days or sooner if the results suggest that cancer could be present. They, of course, also notify your physician.

What's Covered? All group health, sickness or accident policies and group subscribers to health maintenance organizations or fraternal benefit societies that provide hospital or medical/surgical coverage must also provide coverage for mammograms. The minimum coverage required includes all costs associated with a mammogram every year for women 40 years of age and older. The state Medicaid program provides annual screening mammograms for their beneficiaries at any age and diagnostic mammograms when needed. Medicare beneficiaries may receive screening mammograms once a year and diagnostic mammograms whenever medically necessary.

Women who are uninsured or underinsured may be eligible for free mammograms through various programs such as: The Pennsylvania *HealthyWoman Project* through the Pennsylvania Department of Health for women 50 to 64 years (1-877-PA-HEALTH); the Pennsylvania Breast Cancer Coalition's annual *Mother's Day Mammogram* program for women 40 years and older (1-800-377-8828) and the *Mammogram Voucher Program* (1-888-MVP-0505) for women living in Western or Central Pennsylvania.

These groups may also provide follow-up diagnostic services if your mammogram screening signals a need for further examination. Family Planning Councils, local health departments and state health centers—all listed in the blue pages of your phone book—may also provide free mammograms or can refer you to someone who does.

Lumpectomy and breast conserving surgery

What is it? Lumpectomy removes only the lump found in the breast and a surrounding margin of normal tissue. If the removed tissue exhibits cancer cells at its edge (known as the margins), the surgeon may need to remove additional tissue. This may involve a segmental (partial) mastectomy or quadrantectomy (one-quarter of the breast) that removes more breast tissue than a lumpectomy. Radiation therapy is often given as an added precaution to eradicate any remaining cancer cells. This type of surgery is offered in cases of very early stages of cancer as an effort to conserve the breast.

What's covered? Most insurance companies cover a portion or all of this type of surgery. However, because this is often done on an outpatient basis, before you have the surgery, be sure to ask your benefits manager whether the location of your procedure and the physician who is performing it are covered within your network or not. Some companies have actually found it less expensive to cover the costs of a mastectomy (removal of the entire breast) because the lumpectomy is often more time-consuming, and radiation treatments will add to the costs. Medicare does cover lumpectomies and breast-conserving surgery. Your deductible and copay are determined by your plan and whether the surgery is inpatient or outpatient.

Mastectomy

What is it? A mastectomy is the removal of the breast. It is performed when the cancer is widespread and the breast tissue cannot be saved. There are three types of mastectomies: a *simple mastectomy* that removes the breast; a *modified radical mastectomy* that removes the breast and the lymph nodes in the area under your arm; and a *radical mastectomy* that removes the breast, underarm lymph nodes, and muscle located under your breast.

What's covered? Pennsylvania law (*Breast Cancer Reconstructive Surgery Coverage Act, 1997*) requires health insurance policies that provide mastectomy coverage to allow you to receive inpatient care for a length of stay that your treating physician believes is medically necessary. You may also receive home health care within 48 hours after leaving the hospital when your discharge occurs within 48 hours following your admission to the hospital for your mastectomy.

TIP

Before you begin the treatment, be sure to ask your insurance representative and physician whether or not the type of chemotherapy you are being prescribed and where it is being administered to you is covered.

You will be charged whatever copayment, coinsurance, or deductible amounts that are set forth in your policy. These fees must be consistent with what your insurance carrier charges for other benefits under your plan. Medicare covers mastectomies under Part A since this is an inpatient operation.

TIP ✍

While we were going to print with this book, legislation was pending for the HealthyWoman Project to cover mammograms for women 40 years and over instead of 50 years. We feel hopeful that the legislation will eventually pass. So, if you're in your forties, give them a call to see if they are now covering mammograms for women 40 years to 64 years of age.

Reconstruction

What is it? If you have a mastectomy, you may decide that you would like to have reconstructive surgery to recreate your breast. There are two major options for reconstructive surgery: an implant or a muscle flap procedure. The implant, the simpler procedure, involves inserting a saline-filled sac under the chest muscle or an "expander," which is similar to a balloon that a plastic surgeon fills with salt water over an extended period of time.

Muscle flap surgery involves taking flaps of tissue from your skin, fat, and muscle to form a new breast. The most common areas for taking donor tissue are the abdomen, back, and buttocks.

There are two types of muscle flap procedures. In *Attached Flap* (pedicle) surgery, the blood vessels that are attached to the donor tissue remain intact so they continue to receive their own blood supply. The most common procedure of this type is a *TRAM Flap,* using tissue from the abdomen. The other type of flap is a *Free Flap* in which the surgeon detaches the donor tissue from its blood vessels, places it in the chest area, and then carefully sews the cut blood vessels together. This procedure is very specialized and requires longer surgery.

What's covered? You may opt to have reconstructive surgery at the same time as your mastectomy or you may elect to have the surgery later. In either case, Pennsylvania and federal laws protect you: if your insurance carrier covers mastectomies, it must also cover reconstructive surgery related to a mastectomy. This also includes any surgery needed to establish symmetry with your remaining breast. These provisions are covered under the federal *Women's Health and Cancer Rights Act (WHCRA)* of 1998.

WHCRA may not, however, apply to certain "church plans" or "governmental plans," so be sure to check with your employer first to determine whether they fall under either of these categories.

Pennsylvania law (Act 81, 2002) requires that insurance companies place no limit on the time between a mastectomy and the reconstructive surgery. So, if you feel you need more time to consider the surgery after a mastectomy, take it. Even if you decide five or ten years (or longer) after your mastectomy to have the reconstructive surgery, it will be covered, as long as you are under an insurance plan that also covers mastectomies at the time you elect to have reconstructive surgery.

Your insurance carrier may charge you deductibles and coinsurance fees for reconstructive surgery. These fees, however, must be consistent with what they charge for other benefits under your plan. Medicare Part A also covers the surgery as an inpatient procedure.

Lymphedema

What is it? If you have breast cancer surgery that involves removal or radiation of your axillary lymph nodes located in your armpit, it is quite possible that your lymph nodes may not drain as well as they did prior to the surgery. If this occurs, you may develop a condition known as lymphedema, which simply means the build-up of lymph fluid (edema) in the fatty tissues just under your skin. About one in five women develop this condition: they may experience an overall sense of heaviness in the arm, swelling and/ or tightness of the skin.

Treatment for lymphedema can be offered on an outpatient basis by a certified therapist. The treatments may include skin care and hygiene, manual lymph drainage, compression bandaging, therapeutic exercises, compression garments and self-care programs that include the use of pneumatic compression pumps.

TIP ↪

Before you schedule an expensive test (such as a CT or PET scan) that may run into the thousands of dollars, make sure that your plan will cover it. Ask the physician's office prescribing the test to call your company to see whether any restrictions apply.

What's covered? Pennsylvania and federal law requires that those health insurance policies that provide coverage for mastectomies also provide coverage for physical complications including lymphedema. Make sure your physician writes a prescription for the treatment to assure coverage. Medicare also covers most treatments for lymphedema (including compression garments and pumps).

Chemotherapy

What is it? Chemotherapy is a treatment with a combination of drugs whose purpose is to kill cancer cells that may have invaded other parts of your body besides the breast. It is a systemic approach to preventing cancer cells from spreading or returning. The drugs attack the cancer cell's ability to replicate itself. Your oncologist may recommend "chemo" if the cancer has spread to your lymph nodes or if the tumor shows characteristics that the cancer has spread beyond the breast.

What's covered? The cost of chemotherapy varies by the kinds and doses of the drugs that are prescribed. Costs are also affected by how long you'll take the drugs, how often they are given, and where you receive them: at home, in a clinic or office, or in the hospital. Most health insurance policies cover at least a portion of the cost of many kinds of chemotherapy.

Some chemotherapies may be available through clinical trials. (See the clinical trial section of this guide to learn how to apply.) Medicare will cover chemotherapy; however, copayments and deductibles are affected by whether it is performed on an inpatient or outpatient basis. So always find out in advance whether your insurance coverage depends on *where* the treatment is given.

Radiation therapy

What is it? If you've had any type of breast surgery (even a lumpectomy), your physician may decide that radiation is necessary. High-energy particles or waves, such as x-rays or gamma rays, are targeted at cancer cells to destroy their DNA so they won't be able to reproduce themselves. You will be referred to a radiation oncologist who will oversee your treatment.

TIP

Tender Loving Care ("tlc") is a magazine-like catalog that combines helpful articles and information on products for women coping with cancer treatment. The publication features wigs, mastectomy forms, and a large selection of hats and head coverings. There are articles about living with cancer, a section on frequently asked questions, and profiles on real women fighting the disease. The "tlc" website, www.tlccatalog.org, offers a more direct and interactive shopping experience for patients. For a copy of the "tlc" catalog, call 1-800-ACS-2345.

What's covered? Most insurance companies will cover some or all of your radiation treatment. However, before you begin treatment, find out from your insurance carrier whether the place or group where you will receive the treatment is covered under your plan. Your oncologist may be referring you to a group that is considered out of your network, and you could find yourself paying a hefty bill. Medicare will cover radiation; however, copayments and deductibles are affected by whether it is performed on an inpatient or outpatient basis.

Prostheses

What is it? A prosthesis is a device used to artificially replace or substitute for a missing part of the body. If you've had a mastectomy, a "breast form" can offer you a very realistic substitute in both appearance and touch. The form can be worn in your bra or it can be directly attached to your chest with adhesive tape. Breast forms vary in shapes, sizes, materials, and price. They are usually weighted to achieve balance, and you'll find them made from foam, silicone, cotton, and/or spandex fibers. Breast forms can be purchased ready-made, but you may decide to have one specially fitted and ordered just for you. Ask your doctor's office for a list of specialty stores near you that sell breast forms. And here's a tip: during National Breast Cancer Awareness Month (October), many of these supply shops feature sales.

What's Covered? Pennsylvania Law (Act 81 of 2002) requires health insurance policies that provide coverage for mastectomies to also cover prosthetic devices that are needed as a result of a mastectomy and are prescribed by your attending physician. So, yes, breast forms *are* covered as are bras that have built-in pockets to hold the breast form. But before you begin looking for a breast form, be sure to:

- Ask your physician for a prescription for the breast form.

- Ask your insurance carrier whether there are any restrictions on the type or price of a breast form that will be reimbursed.

- Ask your insurance carrier if they pay for new breast forms every few years.

Wigs, according to the law and just about every insurance company, are not considered prosthetic devices. However, some insurance companies will cover the cost of a wig if a woman loses her hair due to chemotherapy. It is worth a call to your insurance carrier to find out. If they don't cover it, check with your local American Cancer Society or the cancer center treating you; they may offer wigs or know of programs that will help if the cost is a financial burden for you.

Bone marrow transplant

What is it? Bone marrow is the spongy tissue found inside bone that produces the body's blood cells: red cells that carry oxygen, white cells that fight infections, and platelets that form clots. The goal of a bone marrow transplant is to empower your body to withstand high-dose chemotherapy that aggressively attacks the cancer cells but also damages normal blood cells in the process. Your new bone marrow helps replenish the damaged blood cells. Transplanted bone marrow comes from either you or a donor whose bone marrow "matches" yours.

What's covered? Most insurance companies require precertification letters justifying the medical necessity for a bone marrow transplant. Be sure to contact your insurer immediately if you and your physician decide that a bone marrow transplant is an option for you. Since there will be a number of screening and matching tests involved prior to a transplant, you'll want to know whether these—as well as the transplant itself—are covered. Medicare does not cover bone marrow transplants as of 2005. In Pennsylvania, the Medical Assistance program does cover bone marrow transplants.

9. SCREENING AND DIAGNOSTIC TESTS: How to tell the difference

You'll likely be undergoing a good number of tests: blood work, x-rays, CT scans, and PET scans to name a few. Some of these tests are preventive, in that you are not showing any symptoms but your doctor wants you to have the procedure to screen for any potential problems. One of the most common breast cancer screening procedures other than breast self-examination is the mammogram. The vast majority of women go through this procedure every year to screen for a possible lump even though there is no appearance of one or of any symptoms of breast cancer. In this instance, the mammogram is a *screening* test.

On the other hand, if the mammogram reveals a lump, your physician may then order a more expensive test such as a CT scan to help him or her better diagnose the nature of the lump. In this instance, the test is *diagnostic*.

Now, what does this have to do with insurance? Depending upon your insurance plan, coverage for a test may be denied if it is considered unwarranted or if the carrier believes that the physician should have used a less expensive test first. For example, if your physician ordered a CT scan *before* you had a mammogram, the insurer might say that you should have been prescribed the less expensive mammogram rather than a very expensive CT scan, which, in this case, was essentially used as a screening device rather than a diagnostic one.

Most insurance plans today encourage screenings because catching potentially life-threatening illnesses early is better for you and less costly for them. Check with your health plan to see what screenings they pay for each year. Medicare does cover mammogram screenings once every 12 months, and a physician's prescription is not required to receive it. Just make sure that the facility performing the mammogram is certified by Medicare.

10. PREAUTHORIZATION
and utilization review

Many plans — and almost all managed care plans — require you to receive approval before you undergo any significant procedure or surgery. This is referred to as preauthorization or precertification. These insurers use a process of "utilization review" in which experts within their system assess whether a specific medical or surgical service is appropriate and/or medically necessary. Never assume that, just because your physician prescribes a procedure or recommends surgery, it will automatically be covered.

If you are in a managed care plan, your Primary Care Physician (PCP) will likely handle this process for you. If you are not in managed care, read your policy to find out whom you call to gain preauthorization approval and under what circumstances.

If you are denied access to a service or procedure that you believe is medically necessary, you can file an appeal with your insurer. See Part V of this guidebook for guidance on how to write a necessary appeal letter.

II. COVERAGE FOR
second opinions

You may be faced with deciding whether you need surgery or choosing one type of surgery over others. Deciding what approach is best for you, especially among the different kinds of mastectomies available today, may be one of the toughest decisions you'll ever make. Getting a second opinion from another physician may be a very wise move. In fact, some insurance plans actually require a second opinion. Before you see a second doctor, ask your insurer if the plan will cover the costs of a second opinion. If you are in a managed care plan, you will likely be referred to another physician but within the plan's network.

Medicare will cover second opinions and will even consider paying for a third opinion if the first and second opinions are not the same.

Pennsylvania's Medical Assistance program also provides coverage for second opinions. If you are enrolled in the ACCESS Plus+ program, you do have a right to a second opinion. According to the program's handbook, you must call your Primary Care Physician (PCP) or the Access Plus+ toll free Helpline at 1-800-543-7633 for a referral if your PCP or a specialist recommends that you have non-emergency surgery and you want a second opinion. The second opinion should provide you with information on the pros and cons of the treatment under consideration. If you are a member of the HealthChoices program, the contractor must provide a second opinion from a qualified health care provider within the network at no cost to the member. If you cannot find a qualified health care provider in the network, they must assist you with finding such a provider outside the network at no cost to you.

12. WHY IT MATTERS WHERE
you receive surgery or a procedure

Be sure to find out whether your insurance plan has any restrictions as to *where* you receive a treatment, procedure, or surgery. Most of the concern will center on whether it is performed at an inpatient setting (usually a hospital) or on an outpatient basis such as clinics, surgery centers, or home health care in your own home. Depending upon what kind of care you are receiving, the plan may decide to reimburse only services provided on an inpatient basis. For example, some new chemotherapy drugs can be taken at home, but the insurance company may reimburse for the treatment only if it is given at an outpatient clinic of a hospital. This also holds true for Medicare.

TIP

Before you begin any type of treatment or have a procedure done, make sure that where you will receive the service doesn't stand in the way of your insurer's paying for it. For example, you may discover that a chemotherapy drug will cost you $2,000 out-of-pocket because you took it at home, but it would be 100 percent covered if you took the same drug at an outpatient clinic. In this case, it's well worth the effort to go to the clinic.

13. GETTING DRUG COVERAGE
when it's <u>not</u> covered by your plan

If your physician prescribes a medication that your insurance plan does not cover and you cannot afford, ask him or her to give you samples or help you apply for a drug assistance program. Some oncologists and cancer centers have a great deal of experience in knowing how to acquire drugs for patients with no financial resources to purchase them. So ask.

TIP 🖎

For drug company sponsored free prescription programs, you will need to take the form to your physician who prescribed the medication and ask for his/her signature along with specific information that may be required by the program. Depending on the eligibility rules, either you or the doctor will need to mail the forms to the drug company sponsoring the benefit.

National assistance programs

Two "one-stop-shop" programs can help you find out whether you qualify for free prescriptions for any condition, not just breast cancer. You can either call their toll free numbers or visit their very easy to use websites. Both groups will provide you with the forms to apply.

The *Partnership for Prescription Assistance* (PPA) is backed by a national coalition of pharmaceutical companies, healthcare providers, and the American Academy of Family Physicians, the NAACP, and a growing number of advocacy associations dealing with diseases.

Here's what it does: PPA helps patients without prescription coverage enroll in more than 275 patient assistance programs (150 offered by the drug companies) and access more than 1,200 medicines, and it advises them on how to contact government programs for which they may qualify, such as Medicaid and Medicare.

The fact that there are hundreds of assistance programs makes tracking them down and dealing with their separate eligibility rules and individual forms stops most people from applying. Using PPA's website and toll free number, however, greatly increases the odds of finding something. The website (www.pparx.org) is very nicely designed and easy to access. There are three different sections: one for doctors, one for caregivers, and one for patients. If you are working for a doctor's office, you can access this site and download forms directly for your patients. To access the program by phone, you can call toll-free at 1-888-4PPA-NOW (1-888-477-2669).

The program is intended to assist people who lack prescription drug coverage and need help paying for their medications. In most cases, this means an income below 200% of the federal poverty level (approximately $19,000 for an individual or $31,000 for a family of three, as of 2005). People who are already enrolled in other publicly and privately sponsored programs that include prescription coverage won't be eligible for assistance. Each of the patient assistance programs available through the *Partnership for Prescription Assistance* has its own eligibility criteria. The PPA single point of access helps you sort through the benefits maze.

Whether you call or go online, you'll need to share some basic information to identify the program(s) for which you may be eligible, so expect to provide your: age, state of residence, zip code, estimated gross annual household income, number of people living in your household, brand name of the prescription medicine you've been prescribed, and, if applicable, any type of health insurance and/or prescription coverage you hold.

You'll learn very quickly which programs you may qualify for, and if you access the program by phone, the program specialist will help fill out the applications and mail them directly to you. If you go online, you'll be able to download, print out, and complete the application.

And how will you get your medications? Depending on the program, the prescription medicines are either sent to your physician's office or to your home. Some patient assistance programs may send you a pharmacy card that you take to your local pharmacy to receive the drug.

The National Council on Aging also offers an excellent free drug benefit assistance service known as *Benefits CheckUpRX* providing access to 250 drug programs including many state and government programs that cover 1,450 drugs. Go to the NCA website at www.benefitscheckup.org. It is an online service only.

State Assistance Programs

Two basic state programs offer prescription assistance: the Department of Aging's PACE and PACENET program for those 65 years and older and the Medicaid prescription assistance program offered by the Department of Public Welfare.

PACE and PACENET

PACE and PACENET offers comprehensive prescription medication coverage to older Pennsylvanians including insulin, syringes, and insulin needles. Neither program covers over-the-counter medicines such as aspirin and cold medicines nor medical equipment. You won't be paying any premiums or monthly fees if you're enrolled in these programs.

Enrollees must be 65 years of age or older and Pennsylvania residents for at least 90 days prior to the date of applying. If you're already enrolled in the Department of Public Welfare's Medicaid prescription benefit, you must stay with that program and NOT apply for PACE.

Eligibility is determined by your previous calendar year's income. For a single person, the total income must be $14,500 or less. For a married couple, the combined total income must be $17,700 or less. If you're accepted, you'll receive a PACE benefit card that you'll present to your pharmacist. You will pay only a $6 copayment for each

generic prescription and a $9 copayment for each brand-name prescription.

PACENET helps seniors with higher incomes who do not qualify for PACE but who still have modest means and are hit with high drug bills. Age, residency, and Medicaid requirements are the same as PACE, but the income limits are higher and—like PACE—are based upon the previous calendar year's income. A single person's total income may range between $14,500 and $23,500 while a couple's combined total income may range between $17,700 and $31,500. Upon qualification, you'll receive a benefit card, but—unlike PACE—you are responsible for a $40 deductible each and every month before the program begins reimbursing for your prescriptions. You will pay an $8 copayment for each generic prescription and a $15 copayment for each brand-name prescription. You cannot apply prescription costs prior to being enrolled in PACENET towards your deductible. You will be paying up to $480 in deductibles for the enrollment year.

PACE does not ask for proof of income when you enroll, however, what you reported to them will be verified with the U.S. Social Security Administration, the IRS, and the Pennsylvania Department of Revenue. Applying is easy. You can go online at www.aging.state.pa.us and click onto PACE/PACENET or call 1-800-225-7223. Enrollment forms are also available at most pharmacies and senior centers.

State Medicaid program

The state Medical Assistance program provides prescription coverage for its enrollees. For more information on this benefit, see Part III, Path 4 of our guide.

Pharmacy discounts

The Pennsylvania Department of Aging provides information about both public and private programs that are available in the state and nation. You do not need to be elderly to take advantage of this excellent service. Call 1-800-955-0989 for The *Pennsylvania Patient Assistance Program Clearinghouse* to learn about drug discount programs that can assist you.

14. HOSPICE

Hospice care brings together medical care, pain management, and emotional and spiritual support for terminal patients and their families. This care is provided in the patient's home when possible or in an inpatient hospice facility with a home-like setting. The mission of hospice staff and volunteers is to address the symptoms of a terminal illness with the intent of promoting comfort and dignity. They are experts at pain management.

Most insurance plans will cover hospice care since it is much less expensive than opting for hospital based or facility-based care. Be sure to review your plan to determine any specific restrictions.

Pennsylvania's Medicaid program also includes a hospice benefit that is similar to the federal Medicare program described below. The state Department of Welfare requires the hospice provider to be certified by the state's Medicaid program and the federal Medicare program.

Medicare does provide a hospice benefit that covers almost all of the costs of caring for a dying person during his or her last six months of life. To qualify for the Medicare hospice benefit:

· You must have Medicare Part A.

· Your doctor and the medical director of the hospice must confirm that you have a life expectancy of less than six months.

· You must agree in writing that you will not pursue any treatments that attempt to "cure" your illness (such as chemotherapy treatments).

TIP ✑

If you are terminally ill, have no insurance, and do not qualify for Medicaid benefits, call the local hospice and ask whether they will provide services. Many charities and foundations make funds available to hospices to assist those without the means to pay. You can find a local hospice by calling the National Hospice Helpline at 1-800-658-8898.

The Medicare hospice benefit covers: skilled nursing services, physician visits, skilled therapy (e.g. physical, speech or occupational), medical social services, nutrition counseling, bereavement counseling, 95 percent of the cost of prescription drugs for symptom control and pain relief, short-term inpatient respite care to relieve family members from care giving, and home care. Medicare does not cover 24-hour round-the-clock care in the home; however, in a medical crisis continuous nursing and short-term inpatient services are available.

Your physician should be able to refer you to a hospice. You can also visit the National Hospice Organization's website at www.nhpco.org and click on a map that will identify the Medicare-certified hospices in your area, call Medicare directly at 1-800-633-4277, or look in the Yellow Pages under Hospices. Here's a list of questions you should ask:

- Are you Medicare-certified? (If not, Medicare will not pay nor will the state Medicaid program).

- Are you a member of any professional organizations or are you accredited?

- Are there certain conditions that patients and families have to meet to enter the hospice program?

- Are you willing to come to the home and conduct an assessment to help us understand whether this is the best option for my family and me?

- What specialized services do you offer such as rehab therapists, family counselors, pharmacists, used equipment?

- What are your polices regarding inpatient care? What hospital(s) do you have a contractual relationship with in the event I would need to go to the hospital?

- Do you require a primary family caregiver as a condition of admission?

- What are the caregiver's responsibilities as related to the hospice?

- What kind of emergency coverage do you offer? Who is on call? Will a nurse come quickly to the home, if needed?

- What out-of-pocket expenses can I expect?

- Will your staff handle all of the paperwork and billing?

- What are your policies on the use of antibiotics, ventilators, dialysis, and/or nutrients given intravenously?

- What treatments are beyond your authority?

INFORMATION FOR YOUR unique circumstances: Six paths of insurance

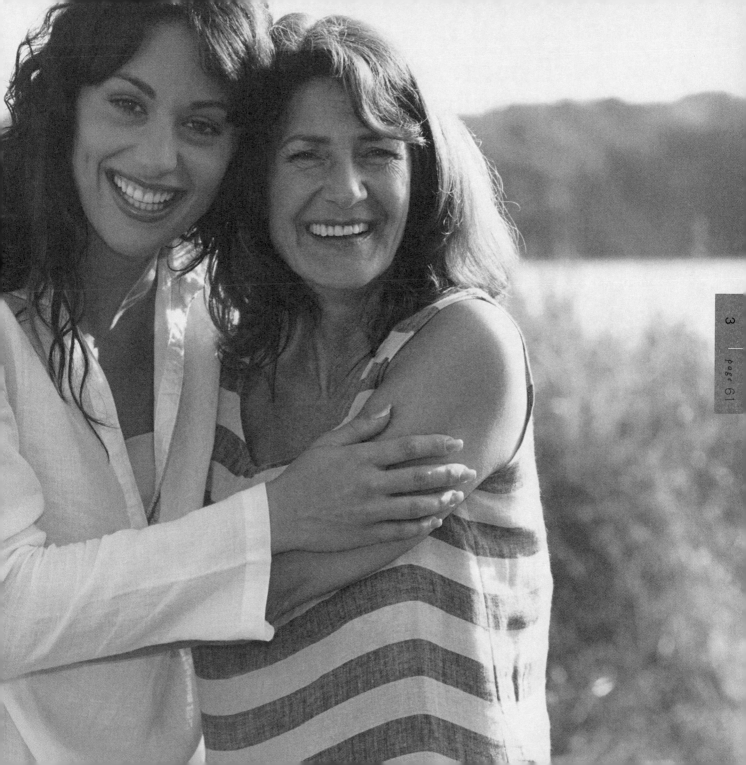

Path 1:
If you're employed

Is your employer self-insured or fully insured?

What's the difference?

Self-insured. In this type of plan, an employer assumes the financial risk of covering its employees by paying medical claims from its own resources. Employers who self-insure control the assets and investments that finance the plan and eliminate paying state taxes on premiums. Large companies tend to self-fund more often than small ones. In some cases, the employer may contract with an insurance company to simply *administer* the program on their behalf. It does not mean, however, that the insurance company administering the program is providing your coverage.

Only federal laws and regulations govern self-funded plans. The law, known as the *Employee Retirement Income Security Act* (ERISA), governs self-insured health plans. Don't be misled by the title into thinking that it applies only to retirees; it governs healthcare coverage, including retirement benefits for working adults.

Fully-insured. If your employer purchases health coverage directly from an insurance company or other underwriter that assumes the full risk for their employees' medical expenses, then it is considered "fully-insured." State laws regulate this type of plan. In this case, the employer pays premiums to the insurance company to provide healthcare benefits to their employees.

TIP ↵

If you ever need to file an appeal on any matter regarding your healthcare coverage, your rights depend upon whether the plan is governed by state law or federal law. To better understand your rights and what laws apply to you, be sure to ask your employer whether your plan is self-insured or fully-insured.

Why this matters to you. The major difference between these two categories is that *self-insured* plans are governed by federal law (ERISA) while fully insured plans are governed by state laws. Another federal law, the Women's Health and Cancer Rights Act (WHCRA), protects employees of self-insured plans with breast cancer. State health insurance laws are traditionally more comprehensive than ERISA, offering greater consumer protection. On the other hand, some self-funded programs tend to offer more generous benefits than fully insured plans.

What every employee needs to know

COBRA: If you should lose or change your job. If you have had health coverage as an employee benefit and you leave your job, voluntarily or not, there is a law known as COBRA (Consolidated Omnibus Budget Reconciliation Act) that will allow you to stay in your employer's group health plan for an extended period of time. *You will, however, be responsible for paying your premium.*

You must meet three criteria in order to qualify for COBRA continuation coverage:

First, you must work for an employer with 20 or more employees. If you work for an employer with 2-19 employees, you may qualify for state continuation coverage.

Second, you must be covered under the employer's group health plan as an employee or as the spouse of an employee.

Third, you must have a qualifying event that will cause you to lose your group health coverage. "Qualifying events" include termination from your job, death of the employed spouse, reduction in hours, and divorce from a spouse.

There are different deadlines you must meet to notify your employer that you want to continue your coverage through COBRA. These deadlines are based upon what kind of event qualifies you. For example, if you terminate your job because of your breast cancer, you need to notify your employer within 30 days that you are electing to receive COBRA coverage. You will be able to receive your coverage for 18 months from the day you resigned from your job. It is not renewable. COBRA coverage is retroactive to the qualifying event, and of course, you will have to pay premiums dating back to this period.

The best way to know which deadline for notification applies to your circumstances is to meet with your Benefits Manager as soon as possible. To learn more about COBRA coverage go to the United States Department of Labor's website at www.dol.gov and enter the keyword *COBRA* at the search function.

Since you will be continuing your coverage, the group insurance plan cannot exclude you due to any pre-existing condition.

You are required to pay for the entire premium. (That includes both the employer and employee share plus a two percent administrative fee.)

If and when you join a new plan, you can keep whatever COBRA continuation coverage you have left during the new plan's pre-existing condition exclusion period.

TIP

The Department of Labor website provides you with details on the law and what your rights are under the Family Medical Leave Act. You can visit the site at www.dol.gov. You can find a sample letter requesting time off based upon FMLA in the Tool Kit section of this book.

Conversion

If you have coverage through an employer's fully insured group health plan and then lose it, you can buy what is known as *conversion* coverage from the company that insured your employer's group plan. You must have been covered under your prior group health plan for at least three months. When you apply, you cannot be covered under a policy with similar benefits or eligible for a similar group or individual health policy plan or Medicare. You must apply within 31 days of being notified.

Conversion policies must meet minimum standards set by state regulations. Don't be surprised, however, to find that your benefits are less generous than what you received before. The insurance company cannot impose a new pre-existing condition exclusion period with your conversion policy. However, you might have to satisfy the portion of any pre-existing condition exclusion period that has not expired from your former health plan.

Chances are, your premiums for the conversion policy will be higher than what you had paid while you were employed; however, they are limited to 20 percent above what you would pay under a similar group policy. You do have the right to renew the policy; it cannot be cancelled because of your breast cancer. This feature is referred to as "guaranteed renewability," but you must be very diligent in paying your premiums.

Family Medical Leave Act (FMLA)

The Family and Medical Leave Act (FMLA) protects workers from losing their jobs when they need time to care for a seriously ill family member or need care themselves. Employers with 50 or more employees must allow their workers at least 12 weeks of unpaid leave for a family member who is seriously ill or for medical leave when the employee is unable to work because of a serious health condition. The law defines family members as the worker's spouse, parent, or child. If you are caring for your in-law or grandparent, the law does not apply. To qualify, you must have worked for the company an average of 24 hours or more per week for at least one year. Your company must give you full health benefits during your leave, and you are entitled to get your old job back or another position with equivalent duties and the same salary and benefits.

Americans with Disabilities Act (ADA)

The Americans with Disabilities Act applies to employers with 15 or more employees. An employer may not discriminate against a qualified individual who has a mental or physical impairment that substantially affects one or more major life activity, such as walking or ambulating in other ways. The Act considers a "qualified individual" as someone who can perform the "essential functions" of a job with or without reasonable accommodation. Employers must provide reasonable accommodations for you as long as these do not impose an undue hardship on the employer. For more information on ADA, go to www.dol.gov or call 1-866-4-USA-DOL. For suggestions on how to write a letter seeking reasonable accommodations needed because of your breast cancer, see the Tool Kit section of this guide.

Annual benefits updates

Every year your employer's health benefit plan administrator should give you an update called a "Summary Plan Description" on what is covered under your health benefits. Always take the time to read it! The requirement to disclose the information surrounding your health insurance coverage and/or retirement plan is covered under federal and state laws, depending upon whether your plan is self-insured or fully-insured. The description will explain what the plan provides in terms of health benefits, how it operates, and how to file claims and appeals among other things. If your plan has changed, you must be informed by either a revised summary plan description or in another document called a "Summary of Material Modifications."

PATH 2: IF YOU ARE
A Medicare beneficiary

As described in Part I of this guide, Medicare provides some level of coverage on nearly all types of surgeries and most treatments related to breast cancer including chemotherapy and radiation therapy. Medicare also offers support for clinical trials.

Below is a brief review of some of the basics on Medicare to assist you in understanding your coverage.

The Basics

Medicare has two distinct parts: Part A and Part B. Medicare Part A helps pay for hospital and facility charges and it is financed primarily by payroll taxes. Part A is sometimes referred to as "Hospital Insurance" and it helps pay for inpatient services, such as inpatient hospital care, coverage for home health care and hospice care, and, if guidelines are met, care in a skilled nursing facility. Part A is generally free for an individual and their spouse who has worked and paid into the Social Security system ("FICA" tax, or for some government employees, it would be a "Medicare" tax) for at least 10 years. Those have not worked and paid into the Social Security system may choose to purchase Part A coverage.

Medicare Part B is financed by Federal general tax revenues and beneficiary premiums. Part B is sometimes referred to as "Medical Insurance" and it helps pay for physician and health care professional services, durable medical equipment, laboratory, ambulance service and supplies. The monthly Part B premium ($78.20 in 2005) is automatically deducted from a beneficiary's Social Security check each month. This Part B premium must continue to be paid even if a person is enrolled in one of the Medicare Advantage plans. Generally for services covered by Medical Part B you will have an annual deductible of $110.00 per year in 2005 after which Medicare Part B will pay for 80% of the Medicare approved amount. This includes covering the costs of rooms, drugs you take while you are a patient in the facility and durable medical equipment (e.g. wheelchairs, hospital beds, walkers) and hospice and blood transfusions.

New options

Recently, Congress renamed the Medicare-plus Choice program – the option to sign-up for managed care plans – as *Medicare Advantage*. You can choose to remain with the traditional or original Medicare plan or opt for managed care plans. In 2006, Medicare beneficiaries can also choose to sign up for even more options such as Preferred Provider Plans (PPOs). You'll need to find out whether these different options are available in your geographic area. If you want to join a *Medicare Advantage* Plan option, you must have Medicare Parts A and B, and cannot have End Stage Renal Disease (permanent kidney failure).

To find out if one of these new plans is available in your area, call Medicare at 1-800-MEDICARE (1-800-633-4227) or visit the website at www.medicare.gov. This is also your direct source for questions about your benefits and Medigap policies offered and approved by Medicare in your area.

Medigap policies (Medicare Supplemental Insurance)

The term Medigap refers to Medicare supplemental insurance. This is private health insurance designed to supplement or fill in the "gaps" of what Medicare does not fully cover. For example, in many instances Medicare will cover 80 percent of a provider's bill while you'll need to pick up the other 20 percent, and that's where a Medigap policy comes in – to pick up, in this example, the other 20 percent.

TIP ↢

Every autumn, the Pennsylvania Department of Aging and the Pennsylvania Health Care Cost Containment Council (PHC4) produce a great handbook comparing different Medicare plans throughout Pennsylvania. Just call the APPRISE program at 1-800-783-7067 to receive a copy or visit the following website to access an interactive copy of the report at www.phc4.org.

You must purchase your own Medigap policy, and insurers selling these plans must meet Medicare guidelines. Depending upon the policy you buy, your Medigap plan may help pay for other costs such as your annual Medicare deductible.

EMPLOYMENT-RELATED RETIREE COVERAGE

If you are retired, you may be able to receive health coverage through your former employer or union. This health coverage may supplement Medicare, but it is not Medigap insurance. Do your homework and carefully compare what your retiree coverage may offer you compared with buying a Medigap policy.

To make your life easier, ask your Medicare participating provider to include your Medigap information on the claim form filed with Medicare. Why? Because then Medicare will send the information on to the Medigap insurer and save you the step. You might see the term "Complementary Crossover," which means that an agreement exists between Medicare and your supplemental insurance company that allows Medicare to automatically send claims to your Medigap insurer after they are processed by Medicare.

Medicare Summary Notices (MSN)

The Medicare Summary Notice (MSN) is a record of services billed to Medicare on your behalf. It provides a complete breakdown of how the claim was billed and processed by Medicare.

The MSN will list the services you received by the provider who provided your treatment. It will list:

- Total billed amount by provider(s).

- Medicare's approved amount for the service(s) performed.

- Amount paid to you or your provider(s).

- Amount you are responsible for paying.

- Deductible information.

- Denial information (if necessary).

You'll also see on the notice the words *"This is Not a Bill"* to alert you not to pay any amount you see on the notice. It is simply a listing of the services you have received from healthcare providers. Be sure to maintain these files as your supplemental insurance company (Medigap) policy provider may need a copy of it to process its portion of the bill.

> **TIP** 〜
>
> *In Pennsylvania, your provider cannot charge you more than the amount Medicare has approved to pay for a service. All providers of healthcare services in Pennsylvania that participate with Medicare must accept what Medicare "assigns" as payment in full. Healthcare practitioners may not charge or collect more than the "Approved Charge" as determined by Medicare. You are still responsible for any coinsurance or deductible.*

Participating providers

A *participating* provider is a healthcare professional who has signed a contract with Medicare in which he or she must accept Medicare's approved amount as payment in full. In other words, the provider has accepted "assignment." Medicare usually pays 80 percent of the approved amount.

TIP ⌒

You can receive information assistance on Medicare, long term care insurance, Medicaid, and Medigap policies free from the Pennsylvania Department of Aging's APPRISE program. Well-trained volunteers, many of whom are available at local senior centers, can help you review your circumstances and the best options available to meet your needs.

To find the APPRISE volunteer nearest you, call 1-800-783-7067.

In Pennsylvania, healthcare professionals who sign-up with Medicare automatically accept what Medicare assigns. Our state is one of the few in the country that has passed a law requiring Medicare providers to accept what Medicare assigns as payment in full.

If you believe a healthcare professional is billing you over what Medicare assigns, you should call the Department of State:

Complaint Office
Bureau of Professional and Occupational
    Affairs
P.O. Box 2649
Harrisburg, PA. 17105
1-800-822-2113 (within Pennsylvania)
1-717-783-4854 (outside Pennsylvania)

Medicare carrier

In Pennsylvania, the Medicare carrier is HGS Administrators (HGSA). Its function is to process claims that your healthcare provider has submitted to Medicare for services provided to you. If you have questions, HGSA suggests that you phone rather than write: there's less potential for misunderstanding questions or responses, and your issues can be resolved much faster than if you wrote. Call HGS Administrators at 1-800-633-4227. HGS also have an excellent consumer website at www.hgsa.com, where you can email a question and receive answers to the most frequently asked consumer questions.

You or anyone calling HGS on your behalf should always be prepared to provide:

- Your complete Medicare number, which is found on your red, white, and blue Medicare card.

- Your full name.

- Your date of birth.

- One additional piece of information (i.e., address).

Federal privacy laws limit the type of information the carrier can share with anyone other than the patient (you). If your family member is calling on your behalf about a specific claim, he or she must have a copy of the Medicare Summary Notice (MSN), and the service representative may discuss only information related to that particular notice. If your representative does not have an MSN, then the carrier will need your verbal permission to release data about your file.

If someone calls frequently on your behalf, you'll need to complete a Release of Medicare Information Form to authorize the carrier to speak to this individual. Ask the service representative how to go about receiving and filing the form.

Path 3: If you have long term care insurance

Most long term care insurance policies offer three levels of care: *Skilled care* requires doctors, nurses, and registered therapists; *Intermediate care* requires trained personnel under the supervision of a doctor or nurse; and *Custodial care* provides non-medical personnel who help with the tasks of daily living. This care can be provided in a long term care facility (nursing home or assisted living) or in your own home, with services provided by home healthcare personnel.

Most companies will send a company nurse to examine you to assess your needs and determine what level of care you need. Your physician will also need to prescribe the level of care he or she believes you need. Some policies may also require a hospitalization prior to receiving home healthcare benefits or nursing home care. Even if you are receiving non-medical senior care, the insurance company may insist that the caregivers work for a licensed home health care agency. Before you sign on with any provider of home health care, ask the insurance company if they have any requirements as to whether the agency is licensed and by whom.

Be sure to check your policy to determine your lifetime maximum benefit and whether a designated break between each payment period is required. Some policies allow you to stop paying your premiums once you start receiving nursing home benefits. When you are admitted to a nursing home, immediately ask your insurance agent whether you can stop paying premiums.

PATH 4: IF YOU HAVE NO INSURANCE

State Medical Assistance Program: Medicaid

Medical Assistance or Medicaid is a program run by the state Department of Public Welfare that provides healthcare coverage for hospital, physician, and prescription services for individuals and families who meet certain income limits and cannot afford health insurance. These income limits change periodically, so the best way to find out whether you and your family qualify is to call or go to your local County Assistance Office (CAO). Feel free to call 1-800-692-7462 to find the office nearest to you.

If your medical expenses are extremely high, you could possibly qualify for Medicaid under the "medically needy" category. Income eligibility limits are determined by subtracting your expenses from your income.

The Medical Assistance program is provided through three options:

1. ACCESS Plus+ is a case management program that operates in 42 counties in Pennsylvania. In this program, you will receive a Primary Care Practitioner (PCP) who will coordinate and manage your care. Because of this feature, the program is also referred to as *"Enhanced Primary Care Case Management."* As an enrollee, you have the right to choose the PCP who will provide your primary care and make referrals to specialists when necessary. Enrollees select a physician who is enrolled with the state's Medical Assistance Program. You may also receive disease management for such conditions as asthma, diabetes, and heart disease. Enrollees receive the quality medical and health care that standard health insurance policies offer. Behavioral health services are accessed through the county Mental Health/Mental Retardation (MH/MR) and Drug and Alcohol (D&A) programs.

2. HealthChoices is a mandatory managed care program that is offered in 25 counties throughout Pennsylvania. If you live in one of these counties, you will automatically be enrolled in this program. As of 2005, these are the counties covered by HealthChoices:

- *Southeast Zone* – Bucks, Chester, Delaware, Montgomery, and Philadelphia counties

- *Southwest Zone* – Allegheny, Armstrong, Beaver, Butler, Fayette, Green, Indiana, Lawrence, Washington, and Westmoreland counties

- *Lehigh/Capital Zone* – Adams, Berks, Cumberland, Dauphin, Lancaster, Lebanon, Lehigh, Northampton, Perry, and York counties

Recipients receive quality medical and behavioral health care similar to what standard health insurance policies offer.

3. Voluntary managed care is offered to enrollees of the ACCESS Plus+ program who would prefer a managed care plan. For an explanation of managed care, please see Part II, 4 of this guide. To find out whether a managed care plan (MCO) is available in your county, call 1-800-692-7462 or visit the Department of Public Welfare's website at www. dpw.state.us and click onto Healthcare Information. As with the other Medical Assistance programs, enrollees receive quality medical and health care similar to what standard health insurance policies offer. Behavioral health services are accessed through the county Mental Health and Mental Retardation (MH/MR) and Drug and Alcohol (D&A) programs. You will receive everything offered in the ACCESS Plus+ program and possibly some additional services. As with all managed care plans, you are assigned a Primary Care Physician and are cared for by healthcare professionals within the plan's network.

Benefits for older people through Medical Assistance

Healthy Horizons

The Healthy Horizons program offers a number of benefits available for people 65 years and older who meet certain income levels. Check with your local County Assistance Office to learn whether you qualify.

Healthy Horizons helps with the payment of your Medicare premiums. Individuals must meet income and resource limits that are based on a percentage of the Federal Poverty Income Guidelines (FPIGs) and are revised annually.

Healthy Horizons includes the following:

Qualified Medicare Beneficiary (QMB – Categorically Needy Program)

If you qualify for this benefit, Medicaid will pay your Medicare Part A and Part B premiums, deductibles, and coinsurance. You will also be eligible for medical coverage through the Medicaid program.

Qualified Medicare Beneficiary (QMB-Medicare Cost-Sharing Program)

Also referred to as Healthy Horizons-Medicare Cost-Sharing, this program pays Medicare Part A and Part B premiums, deductibles and coinsurance for individuals who are eligible.

Specified Low-Income Medicare Beneficiary (SLMB Program)

Individuals who qualify for these benefits are eligible for payment of their Medicare Part B premium only.

PA adultBasic

The adultBasic program provides health insurance for adults who meet certain eligibility requirements and who do not have healthcare coverage. The Pennsylvania Insurance Department contracts with four insurance companies throughout the state that offer basic benefits including preventive care, physician services, diagnosis and treatment of illness or injury, inpatient hospitalization, out-patient hospital services, rehabilitation, skilled nursing care, emergency accident and medical care.

You are eligible if:

· You are between the ages of 19 and 64 years.

· You do not have any other healthcare coverage (including Medicaid or Medicare).

· You have been without health insurance for 90 days prior to enrollment for reasons other than loss of health insurance coverage because you are no longer employed.

· You have been a resident of Pennsylvania for at least 90 days prior to enrollment.

· You have U.S. citizenship or permanent legal alien status.

· You meet certain income limits based on the size of your family. For example, in 2005, if you are a family of four, your income cannot be more than $38,700.

Unlike some other health insurance coverage, adultBasic is available even if you have a history of health problems. Your breast cancer diagnosis will not prevent you from signing up for adultBasic!

You will be responsible for some out-of-pocket expenses. As of 2005, these are:

- $32 per month premium payment.

- $ 5 copayment for each visit to a doctor.

- $10 copayment for each visit to a specialist.

- $25 copayment for each visit to an emergency room unless you are admitted to the hospital.

You can enroll in several ways:

1. Apply online by visiting www.compass.state.pa.us hosted by COMPASS, the Commonwealth of Pennsylvania's Access to Social Services. The secure, online application process is accessible 24 hours a day, seven days a week.

2. Apply by phone by calling 1-800-GO-BASIC, and counselors will start the application process for you over the phone.

3. Apply through the mail by calling 1-800-GO-BASIC, and ask to receive a "paper" application that can be returned in an enclosed postage-paid envelope.

Breast and Cervical Cancer Prevention and Treatment Program

Pennsylvania's *Breast and Cervical Cancer Prevention and Treatment Program* provides coverage for your treatment of breast or cervical cancer, or a precancerous condition of the breast or cervix and any other healthcare need, even if your need is unrelated to your cancer or precancerous condition.

To enroll in the Breast and Cervical Cancer Prevention and Treatment Program, you must have been diagnosed with breast or cervical cancer or a precancerous condition of the breast or cervix and receive a free consultation visit, screening test, or diagnostic test through the *HealthyWoman Project*.

After you have been diagnosed with breast or cervical cancer or a precancerous condition of the breast or cervix and want to find out if you are eligible for the BCCPT Program, you should call the *HealthyWoman Project* at 1-800-215-7494. Here is what you can expect when you call:

- You will be asked several questions relating to your age, household income and insurance coverage to see if you are eligible to enroll.

- If eligible, the *HealthyWoman Project* will assist you in completing Part A (two pages) of the breast and cervical cancer application form.

- You will be asked to have a consultation, screening or diagnostic test for breast or cervical cancer provided by or processed through the *HealthyWoman Project*.

- Your healthcare provider will be asked to complete Part B (one page) of the application form.

TIP ✍

You can still qualify for the Breast and Cervical Cancer Prevention and Treatment Program *even if you have not had a screening or diagnostic test through a non–*HealthyWoman Project *healthcare provider. In this case you must release the results of your diagnostic tests to the* HealthyWoman Project *and receive at least one* HealthyWoman Project *service such as a consult, screen, or diagnostic test.*

- The last step is for you to return the completed form to the *HealthyWoman Project* where you enrolled. This form will be sent to your local County Assistance Office who will contact you for information about your insurance coverage to determine if you are eligible for the treatment program. (You may not be eligible if you currently participate in a group health plan, health maintenance organization, Medicare Parts A & B, Medicaid, Armed Forces insurance, or a state health risk pool).

- In some rare circumstances, you may be eligible even if you have insurance—for example, during a period of exclusion (such as a pre-existing condition exclusion or an HMO affiliation period) for treatment of breast or cervical cancer, or when lifetime limits on all benefits under your plan or coverage are exhausted, including treatment for breast or cervical cancer.

You qualify for the Breast and Cervical Cancer Treatment Program if you are:

- Under age 65 years

- U.S. citizen or eligible non-citizen

- Pennsylvania resident and uninsured or your current coverage is limited in scope (e.g. only dental, vision or long term care) or only covers specified diseases or illnesses of which breast and cervical cancer is not covered.

Community services: Non-profit organizations and volunteers

Information sources. You may be quite surprised to learn how many community services and volunteers are waiting to help you, if you just ask. Regional cancer centers and hospitals employ social workers who are more than happy to share lists of community programs that provide services and programs for women facing breast cancer. Services range from helping with transportation and arranging for child and respite care to support groups that can help you cope with the emotional side of breast cancer. Your local hospitals often offer free educational and health screenings, so just contact the public affairs department to stay current on their community programs and ask them to send you their monthly newsletter announcing their public events and programs.

Support groups. The Pennsylvania Breast Cancer Coalition (PBCC) has identified more than a hundred support groups across the state that provide valuable resources to women and their families facing a breast cancer diagnosis. To find a group near you, call 1-800-377-8828 or visit their website at www.pabreastcancer.org.

Individual support. The American Cancer Society sponsors a *Reach to Recovery* program in which trained volunteers who are breast cancer survivors offer face-to-face or phone support and guidance to women diagnosed with breast cancer. Their goal is to offer emotional comfort by encouraging women and their families to express their feelings, openly talk about fears and concerns, and ask questions from someone who is both knowledgeable and sympathetic. As survivors, they offer hope by sharing their own experience and ability to live a normal and productive life.

To find a group near you go to www.cancer.org and click onto the *Community* navigation bar or call 1-800-ACS-2345. By entering your zip code, you'll get a calendar of local events and learn of social services, the cancer society, legal services, food programs, and welfare office in your area.

Friends Like Me care package. The PBCC provides newly-diagnosed women with a complimentary care package that contains educational publications and brochures as well as some "soft touches" like a pink ribbon pin along with bath and body products when available. *Reading with Friends Like Me* is a resource list compiled by the PBCC of books on such topics as diagnosis and treatment, spirituality/inspiration, and humor — all recommended by survivors.

Look Good...Feel Better. This program is a community-based, free, national service that teaches women cancer patients about beauty techniques to help restore their appearance and self-image after chemotherapy and radiation treatments. The program has three components:

- Group programs. Volunteer beauty professionals lead small groups, usually consisting of 6 to 10 women, through practical, hands-on experience. Women learn about makeup techniques, skincare, nail care, and options related to hair loss such as wigs, turbans, and scarves. Each group program participant receives a free kit of cosmetics for use during and after the workshop.

- One-on-one salon consultations. For patients who are unable to attend a group workshop, a free, one-time, individual salon consultation with a volunteer cosmetologist may be available in their area. These trained beauty experts help each patient address her specific skin, hair, and related appearance needs.

- Self-help materials. These materials are free of charge on request through the *Look Good...Feel Better* toll-free number at 1-800-395-LOOK. You'll receive a 30-minute video entitled "*Just For You: A step-by-step guide to help you look good and feel better during cancer treatment.*" The videotape features cancer survivors and volunteers discussing appearance-related side effects of cancer treatment, as well as detailed skincare information, "how to" makeup tips, wig information, and pointers on head coverings. You'll even learn about nail care. Materials are also offered in Spanish.

To find a program near you or to order the self-help material, call the toll-free number at 1-800-395-LOOK or go to the website at www.lookgoodfeelbetter.org. All cosmetology volunteers attend a four-hour certification class in order to become a *Look Good...Feel Better* volunteer. All cosmetics used in the group program are donated and no specific product is promoted.

Faith-based programs. Many congregations of all faiths offer volunteers who will assist you with respite care, shopping, transportation to appointments, and non-medical home assistance. Many do not even expect you to be a member of their church, synagogue, or mosque. Don't be hesitant in reaching out to them.

Community-based social services. Look in the Yellow Pages of your phone book under "social services" and also in the Blue Pages under "government social service agencies" to identify the local agencies available to you. If you're raising a family, childcare services may also be very helpful to you. If you are 65 years or older, be sure to seek out the services of your local area agency on aging. You can locate it by calling the Eldercare Locator number at 1-800-677-1116. Also, look at the Resources Section of this guide in the "Tool Kit" section.

Path 5: If you buy Insurance Yourself

Blue Cross and Blue Shield plans in Pennsylvania will sell an individual health insurance policy to any resident on a "guaranteed issue basis." This means that the policy can be issued to anyone, regardless of his or her prior medical history. If you are HIPAA-eligible (see Part II of our guide), the Blue Cross and Blue Shield plan operating in your region must offer you a choice of at least two state-approved policies whose benefits are comparable to others they typically sell. One of these policies must offer you comprehensive benefits, and a pre-existing condition exclusion period.

In Pennsylvania, Blue Cross and Blue Shield plans operate in every region:

Region	Blue Cross/Blue Shield Plans
Western Pennsylvania	Highmark Blue Cross Blue Shield.
Northeastern Pennsylvania	Blue Cross of Northeastern Pennsylvania and Highmark Blue Shield
Central Pennsylvania	Capital Blue Cross or Highmark Blue Shield
Philadelphia Area of Eastern Pennsylvania	Independence Blue Cross and Highmark Blue Shield.

While these plans are not required to offer you all of the insurance policies that they have available, the policies that they do offer must comply with requirements set by Pennsylvania law including mandated benefits such as breast cancer screenings.

The plans may require a probationary period before most of the coverage becomes effective. This period cannot exceed 30 days for non-accident-related conditions or six months for certain procedures defined as elective. If you suffer an accidental injury, it will be covered immediately.

The plans may charge a premium during this probationary period even though claims other than for accidental injuries will not be paid during this time. The following list of questions and answers is meant to walk you through the decision to buy insurance yourself.

What about coverage for my breast cancer as a pre-existing condition? If you buy a guaranteed issue policy from a Blue Cross and Blue Shield plan, the policy may impose a pre-existing condition exclusion period, but it cannot exceed 36 months. If you make a claim during the first three years of coverage, Blue Cross and Blue Shield can "look back" for a period of five years to determine whether treatment for the condition was ever recommended or provided to you.

TIP ✌

If you're buying insurance on your own, be sure to find out the insurance company's rating. The A.M. Best Company, Standard & Poor's, and Moody's all rate insurance companies after analyzing their financial records. Publications that list their ratings can be found in the business section of libraries or on each company's website.

If you find that the policy does not meet your needs, you may have a ten-day "free look" period to return the policy and get your money back.

If you buy a non-guaranteed issue policy from a Blue Cross and Blue Shield plan, they can exclude a pre-existing condition by imposing an elimination rider. This is an amendment to your health insurance contract that temporarily or permanently excludes coverage for a health condition, body part, or body system.

What can you expect to pay? Premiums will vary, depending on your family size and type of policy you want. If you buy a *guaranteed issue* individual health insurance policy from a Blue Cross and Blue Shield plan, your premiums will not vary on the basis of your health status.

In contrast, if you buy a *nonguaranteed issue* individual health insurance policy from a Blue Cross and Blue Shield plan operating in Pennsylvania, premiums *can* vary due to age, gender, health status, family size, and other factors.

Can these plans cancel my coverage? Not for reasons related to your health. Your health insurance policy cannot be canceled because you become ill. Guaranteed renewability is required by law and remains in effect as long as you pay your premiums.

Can I buy insurance on a temporary basis? Blue Cross and Blue Shield plans do sell temporary health insurance policies, but they do NOT have to guarantee renewing your policy. They will only cover you for a limited time, such as six months. If you decide to renew coverage when the policy terminates, then you'll have to reapply and there is no guarantee that coverage will be reissued at all or at the same price.

Can I buy health coverage sold by other private insurers? You may be able to find other policies on the open market that will provide you with coverage. However, you may find that they charge higher premiums, modify the benefits by increasing the deductible, or exclude your breast cancer treatment from coverage while still abiding by state and federal laws on exclusions.

What if I am self-employed? If you are self-employed with no other workers, you are not eligible to buy a group health plan on your own; therefore, the laws that protect employers' access to group health plans do not apply to you. If you are self-employed and buy your own health insurance, you are eligible to deduct the cost of your premium from your federal income tax.

What about association plans? You may be able to buy health coverage through a professional or trade association. The laws applying to association health coverage can be different than those for other health plans, so do your research in comparing plans. You may also be able to join another group health plan through a family member.

Path 6: If you have a life insurance policy

If you have a life insurance policy, you may be able to sell it to pay for care that is not covered under other insurance policies that you may have. Viaticals, also known as life settlements, are reserved for people who have experienced a significant decline in health. The term viatical comes from the Latin word, viaticum, which means "provisions for a journey." Essentially, the cash could be used to help pay for the provisions (medical care) for an individual's end-of-life journey.

Many people use the money to pay for medical care that isn't covered under their health insurance and for out-of-pocket expenses. Perhaps, you will need home care, medical equipment, or even non-medical care such as help with preparing meals, transportation to doctor appointments, or child care. There are no requirements on how you use the money.

Your first step is to sit down with your insurance agent and learn all of the details of your life insurance plan. You may have an "accelerated death benefit" provision in the plan that allows the policy owner to receive in advance of his or her death a significant portion or the full amount of the policy death benefit. Under a viatical settlement, no one receives the full 100 percent of the benefit, but it can often be up to 80 percent of the benefit and is usually greater than the cash surrender value of the life insurance policy. Of course, once the insured dies, the family receives nothing.

TIP ✍

Before you do anything, talk with your insurance agent; even if you don't see the terms "accelerated death benefit" in the policy, ask about it anyway.

If the insurance company doesn't offer the accelerated death benefit option and you pursue the viatical route, then:

- Make sure the viatical provider (who makes the offer to buy your policy) and the viatical broker (who shops your life insurance policy and represents you) are licensed by the Pennsylvania Insurance Department. Ask to see the license, or visit the website at www.insurance.state. pa.us, or call 1-717-787-2317.

- Ask what will be the exact amount you will receive upon settlement. (The usual range is about 60 to 80 percent of the face value of the policy.)

- Ask for the details of any fees to be charged for this transaction.

- Ask your tax advisor whether you will have to pay taxes upon settlement. Check with your accountant on the latest state and federal laws that apply.

- Ask that the broker show you all the offers that providers have made to buy your life insurance policy from your broker.

- Find out what type of medical proof you will need (diagnosis, life expectancy) to validate the need for a viatical settlement.

- Determine whether the proceeds will affect your eligibility for Medicaid or other government assistance programs.

Under Pennsylvania law, the Department of Insurance requires brokers and providers to be licensed. The law also provides safeguards for consumers: the broker must disclose the commission to be received from the settlement, your medical condition and identity to buyers must remain confidential, and you must have the right to reverse the settlement up to 15 days after the receipt of payment.

If your life insurance policy has a sizable cash value amount right now, you could consider borrowing against the policy. This may be a smarter move because you won't be losing an average of 20 percent of the face value that viatical companies take. Upon death, your beneficiary can use the policy to pay off the loan and will receive the full face value amount less the borrowed amount plus interest. Interest rates are usually fairly modest, in this instance.

Be sure to find out the current face value of your life insurance policy, and then decide with advice from your accountant or financial planner whether it makes more sense to take out a loan against the policy, take advantage of an accelerated death benefit or sell it outright to a viatical settlement company.

WHEN THE ANSWER IS "NO!" Filing an Appeal & Hospital Billing

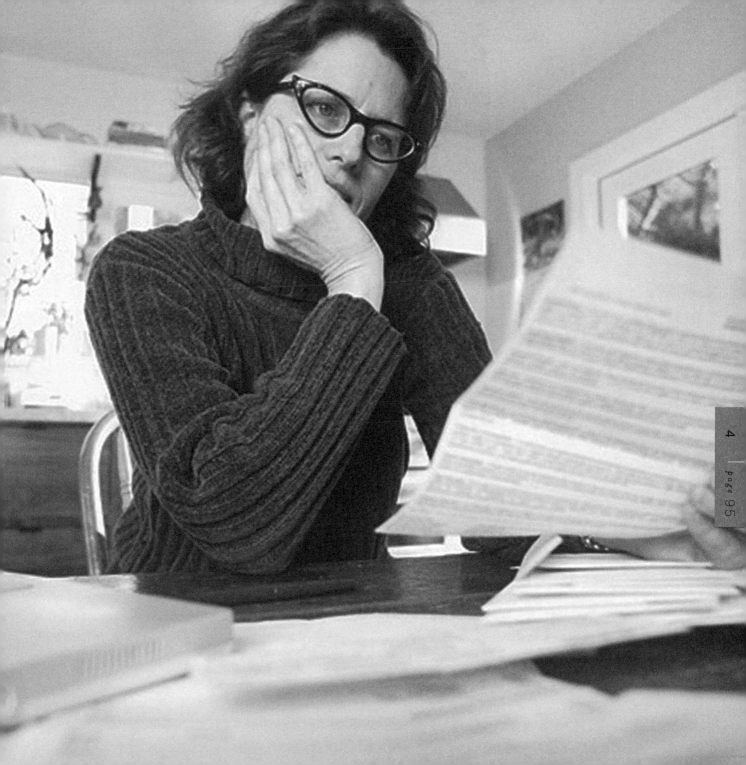

I. DENIALS OF COVERAGE FOR TREATMENT

Your physician may want you to receive treatment or a procedure that requires preauthorization by your insurance company. If you and your physician make the request and it is denied—or if you have already had the treatment assuming it was covered—then you can file an appeal. Here are some tips to help you appeal the denial:

- Immediately phone your insurance company to ask why the claim was rejected. It might be a simple mistake (a clerical or coding error or the need for more information). If it is a simple mistake, it can often be resolved over the phone. You can also ask for a review of the claim over the phone to speed up the process.

- If it is denied because your insurer believes it is NOT necessary, then get a copy of your plan's definition of "medical necessity." Show it to your physician and ask if he or she can demonstrate how your treatment — with further clarification to the insurance carrier — does meet the criteria. Ask your physician to put this in writing so that you can use it to appeal the denial.

- If it is urgent that you receive this care, ERISA-governed plans must make a decision within 72 hours for "urgent care claims" according to federal law.

- If this denial cannot be resolved on the phone and it is not urgent, write a letter to your insurer explaining why the treatment or procedure should be covered. Enclose a copy of the denial notification and the letter from your doctor justifying why the treatment meets the requirements for coverage.

- Request a "Physician Review" from your insurer to have your case reviewed by a doctor of the same specialty as the physician who prescribed your treatment or procedure. Ask the insurer to identify the specific language from your policy that explains why your claim is being denied or paid at a reduced amount. Also, ask for a copy of all medical opinions used in their decision-making to deny your claim. Pennsylvania law requires that the insurer disclose this information to you. On your end, the more physicians who review your case, the more likely you'll find support for your treatment.

- Ask for a case manager, if you are having trouble getting the denial settled. Most companies employ nurse case managers who will act as a liaison between you, your healthcare provider, and the company.

- Go over the time frames cited in your policy (how long the company has to deny your claim and how long you have to file an appeal). Limits for non-urgent cases range from 2 to 45 days; limits for urgent cases range from 24 to a maximum of 72 hours.

- If your insurer will be speaking to your physician to discuss the denial of your treatment, ask if you can be included on the call so that you are able to hear both sides of the issue. During the call, make sure that all parties speak in layman terms!

TIP ✍

Many physicians subscribe to Milliman USA, formerly known as Milliman & Roberts Care Guidelines that identifies and reviews best practices cited in the medical literature and a wide range of clinical settings along with expert medical opinions. If your doctor has access to this resource, ask him or her to provide you with copies of reports that can support your case for the treatment he or she prescribed for you.

- Find out if your insurer is a member of the Utilization Review Accreditation Commission (URAC) at www.urac.org or by calling 1-212-216-9010. This commission sets standards for the healthcare industry and consumer protection guidelines. If you believe that the company violated standards of utilization review, let the URAC know.

- If you've received a denial for a procedure that has already been performed, your appeal letter must include as much medical back up as possible to justify the treatment or procedure. Here's what you need: a *"Medical Necessary Appeal Letter"* from the physician who treated you and also the physician who may have referred you to him or her; medical literature that is peer-reviewed (analyzed by other physicians) that supports your treatment; a timeline of what steps led up to the treatment that is being denied (such as less invasive procedures that were tried first, ineffective treatment or complications you experienced from prior treatment); and any medical evidence that shows that any other procedure will be ineffective.

Complaint or grievance? Pennsylvania law creates a distinction between grievances and complaints. A *grievance* is a request to conduct a review of a covered health service that was denied on the basis of medical necessity or appropriateness. A *complaint* addresses more generalized issues such as how the plan operates, quality of care or service problems, or a dispute over benefits coverage.

Health plans usually determine whether your issue is a grievance or a complaint.

If you file a *grievance* and it is not satisfactorily resolved, you may request a review of your case by an independent Utilization Review Organization (URO).

If your *complaint* is not satisfactorily resolved, you may appeal to the Pennsylvania Insurance Department by sending a copy of your complaint with a request to help resolve the issue. You can file a complaint online at www.insurance.state.pa.us, call the Insurance Department's Office at 1-877-881-6388, or write to one of the Pennsylvania Insurance Department's regional offices:

HARRISBURG

Room 1321 Strawberry Square
Harristown State Office Bldg. #1
Harrisburg, PA 17120
Phone: 1-717-787-2317
Fax: 1-717-787-8585

PHILADELPHIA

Room 1701 State Office Bldg.
1400 Spring Garden Street
Philadelphia, PA 19130
Phone: 1-215-560-2630
Fax: 1-215-560-2648

PITTSBURGH

Room 304 State Office Bldg.
300 Liberty Avenue
Pittsburgh, PA 15222
Phone: 1-412-565-5020
Fax: 1-412-565-7648

For complaints or grievances with managed care plans, call the Bureau of Managed Care, Department of Health, at 1-888-466-2787.

Appeals with Medical Assistance programs

If you have been denied a treatment or procedure, given a lesser benefit, or you disagree with action taken regarding your care through your Medical Assistance HealthChoices or fee-for-service plan, you have the right to appeal the decision. There are three levels of the grievance process plus a fair hearing. If you are currently receiving the service or benefit, it's wise to appeal within 10 days so as to continue the service throughout the appeals process.

For more information on appealing denials, terminations, or reductions of coverage/benefits, contact the *Pennsylvania Health Law Project* by calling 1-800-274-3258 or visit the website at www.phlp.org.

Appeals with Medicare

You have the right to appeal any decision regarding Medicare services whether you are enrolled in the original Medicare plan or in a Medicare managed care plan. If Medicare denies payment for a treatment, procedure, service, or item you have received or for one that you believe you need, you can appeal.

If you think that waiting for a decision about a treatment or service could seriously harm your health, ask the plan for an urgent decision. The plan must respond within 72 hours.

If you do not agree with a denial of a claim or the amount paid on the claim, you have 120 days from the date of finalization to request a review. According to the Centers for Medicare and Medicaid Services (CMS), you must include three items in your appeal:

- A copy of your Medicare Summary Notice (MSN).

- A letter explaining why you want this review. (You may write the reason for the review on the MSN. You'll find Appeals Information located on the last page of your MSN.)

- Medical information that supports the rationale for the treatment from the physician or provider who performed the service or treatment that was denied. Types of records include operative notes, admission and discharge records, order sheets, pathology reports and/or academic journal articles that support the treatment.

If you are unable to request the appeal on your own, you may appoint a representative during any point in the appeals process. You'll need to complete an "Appointment of Representative" form that can be provided to you by calling 1-800-MEDICARE.

In Pennsylvania, if you disagree with a quality of health care decision, such as a denial of care or being told that you need to be discharged from the hospital sooner than you believe is in your best interest, call *Quality Insights* at 1-800-322-1914 to review your case. If this is a hospital discharge dispute, you may be able to stay in the hospital at no charge during the review since the hospital cannot force you to leave before a decision is made.

Quality Insights reviews quality of care complaints on behalf of Medicare beneficiaries in the following healthcare settings:

- Hospital (including psychiatric) or hospital emergency department

- Skilled nursing or rehabilitation facility

- Ambulatory surgery center

- Doctor's office

- Home health agency

If you want to report a poor quality of care experience, you may write a complaint letter detailing the situation and identifying the name of the facility and provider and send it to:

Quality Insights of Pennsylvania
Attn: Review Services
2601 Market Place Street, Suite 320
Harrisburg, PA 17110

2. HOSPITAL BILLING:
Watch for mistakes

Nothing is really standardized when it comes to medical billing — in hospitals, doctor's offices, surgery suites, or even pharmacies. Experts contend that eight out of ten bills contain errors that cause consumers to pay thousands of dollars in out-of-pocket expenses from hospital stays. If your hospital does not send you an itemized bill, you may have to request one by calling their billing department.

Don't be lulled into a false sense of security by thinking that if your insurance company pays your hospital bill that you are free and clear. Not really. Your insurance policy does have a lifetime cap, and billing errors that are paid by your insurance chips away at that cap. If you are ever faced with an extended hospital stay or a catastrophic illness, you'll find yourself invading your life savings if you've exceeded the cap. Medical debt is the second most common reason why Americans file bankruptcy and eight of ten have health insurance!

Here's our "Top Dozen" list of mistakes to watch for:

1. Charging for the day of discharge. Most insurance plans do not allow hospitals to charge for the day you leave the hospital.

2. Charging for a private room when you had a semi-private room or if you were given a private room because no semi-private was available.

3. Charging for medications you didn't receive or refused or charging you for the high-priced brand when your doctor prescribed a generic.

4. Charging for the same procedure or service twice, known as "double billing."

5. Charging for tests that are grouped under a broad category like *blood work* or *miscellaneous*. Always ask for tests to be itemized.

6. Charging for services that your doctor did not order or that may have been scheduled but later cancelled.

7. Charging for a test twice because it was administered incorrectly the first time or the first set of test results was misplaced.

8. Charging for personal items that are usually included in the room charge like those nifty slipper socks, toothbrushes, lotions, and combs.

9. Charging for physician services on the hospital bill when the doctor (such as an anesthesiologist or radiologist) sends you a separate bill for the same service.

10. Charging excessive amounts due to a clerical mistake made by entering the wrong code for a service or procedure.

11. Charging for more operating room time than was used for your surgery. Check your anesthesia record that states when your surgery began and ended.

12. Charging for a more serious diagnostic condition than what your doctor diagnosed, resulting in more costly procedures and an inflated reimbursement rate to the hospital known as "upcoding."

If you suspect a mistake, first call the hospital's billing department and explain the situation. If it isn't resolved over the phone, write a letter detailing the mistake(s) and send it to the hospital. Immediately call your insurance plan, go over the bill with your account representative, and ask where to send a copy of your letter. Keep records of the individuals you talked to, when and what you discussed. Do not wait around. Many hospitals will send your unpaid bill to a collection agency within 90 days, and that can affect your credit rating.

If your hospital bill is very complicated or you feel you need help, you can find medical bill reviewer/recovery consultants who will review your bills, identify mistakes, and handle the paperwork for you between the hospital and your insurer. Often they are paid a percentage of the amount they saved you, which can run as high as 50 percent. The *Alliance of Claims Assistance Professionals* at 1-877-275-8765 (web page at www.claims. org) can give you a referral as can the *Medical Billing Advocates of America* at 1-540-387-5870 (www.billadvocates.com). If you are over 60 years of age, you can also ask an APPRISE volunteer to help you; they are trained by state Insurance and Department of Aging experts and can often be found at your local senior center. If all else fails, the Pennsylvania Attorney General's Health Care Section (1-877-888-4877) may be of assistance.

TOOL KIT

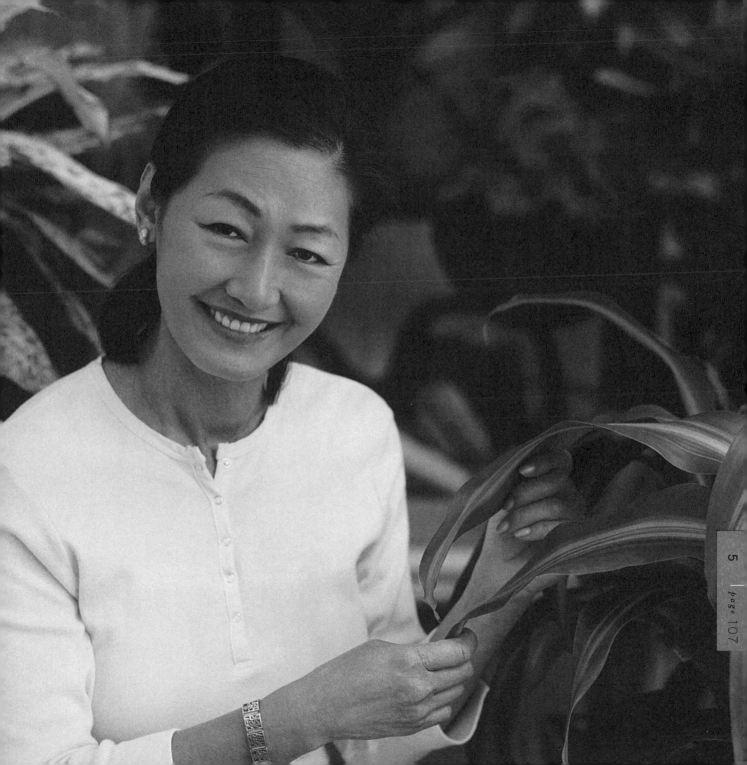

PART V: Tool Kit

A. Insurance questions: Master Check List

B. Sample Letters (How to write them)

- Reasonable accommodations for ADA

- Family Medical Leave Act request

- Medical Necessary Appeal letter

C. Resources (1-800 phone numbers, addresses, websites of breast cancer resources especially relevant to financial and insurance issues)

D. Glossary of insurance terms

INSURANCE QUESTIONS
Master Check List

PA BREAST CANCER COALITION

To prevent future problems regarding coverage for your care, be sure you have the answers to these questions. Use them as a guide as you review your benefit plan and when you talk to your Benefits Manager.

QUESTION	✓
Is my plan self-insured or fully-insured? • *See Part III, Path 1 of our guide to know what this means for you.*	
What kind of plan do I have? (e.g. HMO, Fee-for-service, PPO)	
What are the preauthorization requirements for treatment procedures and/or surgery?	
What are the exclusions of my plan? In other words, what isn't covered?	
Are second opinions covered? • *What procedures do I follow to get one?*	
What is my coinsurance and deductible? • *Does it vary for different treatments and or procedures? (e.g. mental health coverage)*	
Is there a maximum amount of out-of-pocket expenses per year that I am responsible for and then you pick up the rest?	
How is "pre-existing condition" defined?	
If in a managed care plan: • *How can I get a referral to specialists outside of the network?* • *How do I submit an Out-of-Network claim?*	

QUESTION	✓
Are there policy maximums on medical care? Mental health care?	
What are the procedures for filing an appeal? • *Are there timeframes that must be followed?*	
What procedures do I follow to participate in a clinical trial?	
Are there stipulations as to where I receive chemotherapy, surgery or a procedure? (e.g. inpatient at a hospital vs. a free-standing center, doctor's office or at home).	
What is my lifetime benefit amount?	

Insurance Related Resources

PA Department of Insurance

Regional Consumer Office:
1-877- 881-6388
adultBasic Health Insurance Program:
1-800-GO-BASIC
www.insurance.state.pa.us

Social Security Administration

1-800-772-1213
www.ssa.gov

U.S. Department of Labor

Philadelphia Regional Office
1-215-861-4818
For Department of Labor publications:
1-866-444-3272
www.dol.gov/dol/pwba

PA Department of Health

HealthyWoman Project: Breast and
Cervical Cancer Prevention and
Treatment Program
1-877-PA-HEALTH
www.health.state.pa.us

PA Department of Public Welfare

Medicaid & Helpline: 1-800-692-7462
Healthy Horizons: 1-800- 842-2020
www.dpw.state.pa.us

PA Department of Aging

PACE/PACENET: 1-800-225-7223
APPRISE Insurance Counseling:
1-800-783-7067

Long Term Care Helpline

1-866-286-3636
www.aging.state.pa.us

Internal Revenue Service (IRS)

The Federal Health Coverage Tax Credit
(HCTC): 1-866-628-4282
www.irs.gov/individuals/index.html

Medicare

1-800-633-4227
www.medicare.gov
For easy to understand explanation of your
Medicare rights go to:
www.medicarerights.org

US Equal Employment Opportunity Commission

Provides American with Disabilities Act guidance:
1-800-669-4000
www.eeoc.gov

Patient Advocate Foundation

For state by state financial resource guides:
1-800-532-5274
www.patientadvocate.org
For assistance with copays for drugs:
1-866- 512-3861\www.copays.org

Glossary of Health Insurance Terms for Consumers[1]

This glossary is a general guide to terms frequently used discussing health insurance; however, these definitions may not be the same as those detailed in your insurance policy or as defined by applicable state or federal law. Consult how terms are defined by your insurance policy because these and changes to state and federal law will apply and may affect the definitions used in this glossary.

A

Actuary: A mathematician working for a health insurance company responsible for determining what premiums the company needs to charge based in large part on claims paid verses amounts of premium generated. Their job is to make sure a block of business is priced to be profitable.

Admitting Privileges: The right granted to a doctor to admit patients to a particular hospital.

Advocacy: Any activity done to help a person or group to get something the person or group needs or wants.

Affiliation Period: The time an HMO may require you to wait after you enroll and before your coverage begins. HMOs that require an affiliation period cannot exclude coverage of pre-existing conditions. Premiums cannot be charged during HMO affiliation periods. See also HMO.

---

[1] Reprinted with permission from www.healthinsurance.org and the Georgetown University Health Policy Institute 2004.

Agent: Licensed salesperson who represents one or more health insurance companies and presents their products to consumers.

Association: A group. Associations can often offer individual health insurance plans specially designed for their members.

B

Benefit: Amount payable by the insurance company to a claimant, assignee, or beneficiary when the insured suffers a loss.

Brand-name drug: Prescription drugs marketed with a specific brand-name by the company that manufactures it, usually the company which develops and patents it. When patents run out, generic versions of many popular drugs are marketed at lower cost by other companies. Check your insurance plan to see if coverage differs between brand-name and their generic twins.

Broker: Licensed insurance salesperson who obtains quotes and plan from multiple sources of information for clients.

C

Capitation: Capitation represents a set dollar limit that you or your employer pay to a health maintenance organization (HMO), regardless of how much you use (or don't use) the services offered by the health maintenance providers. (Providers is a term used for health professionals who provide care. Usually providers refer to doctors or hospitals. Sometimes the term also refers to nurse practitioners, chiropractors and other health professionals who offer specialized services.)

Carrier: The insurance company or HMO offering a health plan.

Case Management: Case management is a system embraced by employers and insurance companies to ensure that individuals receive appropriate, reasonable health care services.

Certificate of Insurance: The printed description of the benefits and coverage provisions forming the contract between the carrier and the customer. Discloses what it covered, what is not, and dollar limits.

Claim: A request by an individual (or his or her provider) to an individual's insurance company for the insurance company to pay for services obtained from a health care professional.

COBRA: Federal legislation that lets you, if you work for an insured employer group of 20 or more employees, continue to purchase health insurance for up to 18 months if you lose your job or your coverage is otherwise terminated. For more information, visit the Department of Labor. The term stands for Consolidated Omnibus Budget Reconciliation Act.

Coinsurance: Coinsurance refers to money that an individual is required to pay for services, after a deductible has been paid. In some health care plans, coinsurance is called "copayment." Coinsurance is often specified by a percentage. For example, the employee pays 20 percent toward the charges for a service and the employer or insurance company pays 80 percent.

Continuous Coverage: Health insurance coverage that is not interrupted by a break of 63 or more days in a row. Employer waiting periods and HMO affiliation periods do not count as gaps in health insurance coverage for the purpose of determining if coverage is continuous. See also Creditable Coverage.

Conversion Policy: Your right to convert your policy to an individual health plan when leaving a fully insured group health plan in Pennsylvania. You will not face a new pre-existing condition exclusion period. There are limits on what you can be charged for conversion policies.

Copayment: Copayment is a predetermined (flat) fee that an individual pays for health care services, in addition to what the insurance covers. For example, some HMOs require a $10 "copayment" for each office visit, regardless of the type or level of services provided during the visit. Copayments are not usually specified by percentages.

Creditable Coverage: Health insurance coverage under any of the following; a group health plan, an individual health plan, Medicare, Medicaid, CHAMPUS (health coverage for military personnel, retirees, and dependents), the Federal Employees Health Benefits Program, Indian Health Service, the Peace Corps, or a state health insurance high risk pool.

Credit for Prior Coverage: This may or may not apply when you switch employers or insurance plans. A pre-existing condition waiting period met while you were under an employer's (qualifying) coverage can be honored by your new plan, as long as any interruption in the coverage between the two plans meets state guidelines.

D

Deductible: The amount an individual must pay for health care expenses before insurance (or a self-insured company) covers the costs. Often, insurance plans are based on yearly deductible amounts.

Denial of Claim: Refusal by an insurance company to honor a request by an individual (or his or her provider) to pay for health care services obtained from a health care professional.

Dependents: Spouse and/or unmarried children (whether natural, adopted or step) of an insured person.

E

Effective Date: The date your insurance is to actually begin. You are not covered until the policies effective date.

Elimination Rider: A feature permitted in a individual health insurance policy that permanently excludes coverage for a health condition, body part, or body system.

Enrollment Period: The period during which all eligible employees and their dependents can sign up for coverage under an employer group health plan. Besides permitting workers to elect health benefits when first hired, many employers and group health insurers hold an annual enrollment period, during which all eligible employees can enroll in or change their health coverage

Employee Assistance Programs (EAPs): Mental health counseling services that are sometimes offered by insurance companies or employers. Typically, individuals or employers do not have to directly pay for services provided through an employee assistance program.

Exclusions: Medical services that are not covered by an individual's insurance policy.

Explanation of Benefits: The insurance company's written explanation to a claim, showing what they paid and what the client must pay.

F

Family and Medical Leave Act (FMLA): A federal law that guarantees up to 12 weeks of job protected leave for certain employees when they need to take time off due to serious illness, to have or adopt a child, or to care for another family member. When you qualify for leave under FMLA, you continue coverage under your group health plan.

Fully Insured Group Health Plan: Health insurance purchased by an employer from an insurance company. Fully insured health plans are regulated by the state of Pennsylvania. See also Self-Insured Group Health Plans.

G

Generic Drug: A "twin" to a "brand-name drug" once the brand-name company's patent has run out and other drug companies are allowed to sell a duplicate of the original. Generic drugs are less expensive, and most prescription and health plans reward clients for choosing generics.

Group Insurance: Coverage through an employer or other entity that covers all individuals in the group.

Group Health Plan: Health insurance (usually sponsored by an employer, union or professional association) that covers at least 2 employees, or the self-employed. See also Fully Insured Group Health Plan, Self-Insured Group Health Plan.

Guaranteed Issue: A requirement that health plans must permit you to enroll regardless of your health status, age, gender, or other factors that might predict your use of health services. All health plans sold to small employers in Pennsylvania are guaranteed issue.

Guaranteed Renewability: A feature in health plans that means your coverage cannot be canceled because you get sick. HIPAA requires certain health plans to be guaranteed renewable. Your coverage can be canceled, however, for other reasons unrelated to your health status.

H

Health Coverage Tax Credit (HCTC): The Health Coverage Tax Credit (HCTC) is a program that can help pay for nearly two-thirds of eligible individuals' health plan premiums. In general, in order to be eligible for the health coverage tax credit, you must be 1) receiving Trade Readjustment Allowance benefits (TRA), or 2) will receive TRA benefits once your unemployment benefits are exhausted, or 3) receiving benefits under the Alternative Trade Adjustment Assistance (ATAA) program, or 4) aged 55 or older and receiving benefits from the Pension Benefit Guaranty Corporation (PBGC).

Health Maintenance Organizations (HMOs): Health Maintenance Organizations represent "prepaid" or "capitated" insurance plans in which individuals or their employers pay a fixed monthly fee for services, instead of a separate charge for each visit or service. The monthly fees remain the same, regardless of types or levels of services provided. Services are provided by physicians who are employed by, or under contract with, the HMO. HMOs vary in design. Depending on the type of the HMO, services may be provided in a central facility or in a physician's own office (as with IPAs.)

Health Status: Refers to your medical condition (both physical and mental illnesses), claims experience, receipt of health care, medical history, genetic information, evidence of insurability (including conditions arising out of acts of domestic violence), and disability.

HIPAA: A Federal law passed in 1996 that allows persons to qualify immediately for comparable health insurance coverage when they change their employment or relationships. It also creates the authority to mandate the use of standards for the exchange of health care data and specifies the types of measures required to protect the security and privacy of personally identifiable health care. Full name is "The Health Insurance Portability and Accountability Act of 1996."

I

Indemnity Health Plan: Indemnity health insurance plans are also called "fee-for-service." These are the types of plans that primarily existed before the rise of HMOs, IPAs, and PPOs. With indemnity plans, the individual pays a pre-determined percentage of the cost of health care services, and the insurance company (or self-insured employer) pays the other percentage. For example, an individual might pay 20 percent for services and the insurance company pays 80 percent. The fees for services are defined by the providers and vary from physician to physician. Indemnity health plans offer individuals the freedom to choose their health care professionals.

Independent Practice Associations: IPAs are similar to HMOs, except that individuals receive care in a physician's own office, rather than in an HMO facility.

In-Network: Providers or health care facilities which are part of a health plan's network of providers with which it has negotiated a discount. Insured individuals usually pay less when using an In-Network provider, because those networks provide services at lower cost to the insurance companies with which they have contracts.

L

Lifetime Maximum Benefit (or Maximum Lifetime Benefit): The maximum amount a health plan will pay in benefits to an insured individual during that individual's lifetime.

Limitations: A limit on the amount of benefits paid out for a particular covered expense, as disclosed on the Certificate of Insurance.

Long-Term Care Policy: Insurance policies that cover specified services for a specified period of time. Long-term care policies (and their prices) vary significantly. Covered services often include nursing care, home health care services, and custodial care.

Long-term Disability Insurance: Pays an insured a percentage of their monthly earnings if they become disabled.

Look Back: The maximum length of time, immediately prior to enrolling in a health plan, that can be examined for evidence of pre-existing conditions.

LOS: LOS refers to the length of stay. It is a term used by insurance companies, case managers and/or employers to describe the amount of time an individual stays in a hospital or inpatient facility.

M

Managed Care: A medical delivery system that attempts to manage the quality and cost of medical services that individuals receive. Most managed care systems offer HMOs and PPOs that individuals are encouraged to use for their health care services. Some managed care plans attempt to improve health quality by emphasizing prevention of disease.

Maximum Dollar Limit: The maximum amount of money that an insurance company (or self-insured company) will pay for claims within a specific time period. Maximum dollar limits vary greatly. They may be based on or specified in terms of types of illnesses or types of services. Sometimes they are specified in terms of lifetime, sometimes for a year.

Medicaid: A program providing comprehensive health insurance coverage and other assistance to certain low-income Pennsylvanians. All other states have Medicaid programs, too, though eligibility levels and covered benefits will vary. This may also be referred to as Medical Assistance.

Medigap Insurance Policies: Medigap is private health insurance designed specifically to supplement Medicare benefits by filling in some of the gaps in Medicare coverage. Some examples of gaps in Medicare coverage are deductibles, coinsurance and non-covered services. Medigap coverage varies depending upon the terms of the Medigap policy. Some Medigap policies provide coverage for Medicare's deductibles and most pay the hospital and medical coinsurance amounts. These policies are designed to pay for some of the costs that Medicare does not cover.

Multiple Employer Trust (MET): A trust consisting of multiple small employers in the same industry, formed for the purpose of purchasing group health insurance or establishing a self-funded plan at a lower cost than would be available to each of the employers individually.

N

Network: A group of doctors, hospitals and other health care providers contracted to provide services to insurance companies customers for less than their usual fees. Provider networks can cover a large geographic market or a wide range of health care services. Insured individuals typically pay less for using a network provider.

O

Open-ended HMOs: HMOs which allow enrolled individuals to use out-of-plan providers and still receive partial or full coverage and payment for the professional's services under a traditional indemnity plan.

Out-of-Plan (Out-of-Network): This phrase usually refers to physicians, hospitals or other health care providers who are considered nonparticipants in an insurance plan (usually an HMO or PPO). Depending on an individual's health insurance plan, expenses incurred by services provided by out-of-plan health professionals may not be covered, or covered only in part by an individual's insurance company.

Out-Of-Pocket Maximum: A predetermined limited amount of money that an individual must pay out of their own savings, before an insurance company or (self-insured employer) will pay 100 percent for an individual's health care expenses.

Outpatient: An individual (patient) who receives health care services (such as surgery) on an outpatient basis, meaning they do not stay overnight in a hospital or inpatient facility. Many insurance companies have identified a list of tests and procedures (including surgery) that will not be covered (paid for) unless they are performed on an outpatient basis. The term outpatient is also used synonymously with ambulatory to describe health care facilities where procedures are performed.

P

Plan Administration: Supervising the details and routine activities of installing and running a health plan, such as answering questions, enrolling individuals, billing and collecting premiums, and similar duties.

Pre-Admission Certification: Also called precertification review, or pre-admission review. Approval by a case manager or insurance company representative (usually a nurse) for a person to be admitted to a hospital or inpatient facility, granted prior to the admittance. Pre-admission certification often must be obtained by the individual. Sometimes, however, physicians will contact the appropriate individual. The goal of pre-admission certification is to ensure that individuals are not exposed to inappropriate health care services (services that are medically unnecessary).

Pre-Admission Review: A review of an individual's health care status or condition, prior to an individual being admitted to an inpatient health care facility, such as a hospital. Pre-admission reviews are often conducted by case managers or insurance company representatives (usually nurses) in cooperation with the individual, his or her physician or health care provider, and hospitals.

Pre-admission Testing: Medical tests that are completed for an individual prior to being admitted to a hospital or inpatient health care facility.

Pre-existing Conditions: A medical condition that is excluded from coverage by an insurance company, because the condition was believed to exist prior to the individual obtaining a policy from the particular insurance company. For Group Health Plans the look back period will usually be within the six month period immediately preceding enrollment in a plan. For Individual Health Plans the look back period is usually within a five-year period immediately preceding enrollment in a plan.

Preferred Provider Organizations (PPOs): You or your employer receive discounted rates if you use doctors from a pre-selected group. If you use a physician outside the PPO plan, you must pay more for the medical care.

Primary Care Provider (PCP): A health care professional (usually a physician) who is responsible for monitoring an individual's overall health care needs. Typically, a PCP serves as a "quarterback" for an individual's medical care, referring the individual to more specialized physicians for specialist care.

Provider: Provider is a term used for health professionals who provide health care services. Sometimes, the term refers only to physicians. Often, however, the term also refers to other health care professionals such as nurse practitioners, chiropractors, physical therapists, and others offering specialized health care services.

R

Reasonable and Customary Fees: The average fee charged by a particular type of health care practitioner within a geographic area. The term is often used by medical plans as the amount of money they will approve for a specific test or procedure. If the fees are higher than the approved amount, the individual receiving the service is responsible for paying the difference. Sometimes, however, if an individual questions his or her physician about the fee, the provider will reduce the charge to the amount that the insurance company has defined as reasonable and customary.

Rider: A modification made to a Certificate of Insurance regarding the clauses and provisions of a policy (usually adding or excluding coverage).

Risk: The chance of loss, the degree of probability of loss or the amount of possible loss to the insuring company. For an individual, risk represents such probabilities as the likelihood of surgical complications, medications' side effects, exposure to infection, or the chance of suffering a medical problem because of a lifestyle or other choice. For example, an individual increases his or her risk of getting cancer if he or she chooses to smoke cigarettes.

S

Second Opinion: It is a medical opinion provided by a second physician or medical expert, when one physician provides a diagnosis or recommends surgery to an individual. Individuals are encouraged to obtain second opinions whenever a physician recommends surgery or presents an individual with a serious medical diagnosis.

Second Surgical Opinion: These are now standard benefits in many health insurance plans. It is an opinion provided by a second physician, when one physician recommends surgery or a procedure to an individual.

Self-Insured Group Health Plans: Plans set up by employers who set aside funds to pay their employees' health claims. Because employers often hire insurance companies to administer these plans, they may look to you just like fully insured plans. Employers must disclose in your benefits information whether an insurer is responsible for funding, or for only administering the plan. If the insurer is only administering the plan, it is self-insured. Self-insured plans are regulated by the U.S. Department of Labor, not by Pennsylvania.

Short-Term Disability: An injury or illness that keeps a person from working for a short time. The definition of short-term disability (and the time period over which coverage extends) differs among insurance companies and employers. Short-term disability insurance coverage is designed to protect an individual's full or partial wages during a time of injury or illness (that is not work-related) that would prohibit the individual from working.

Short-Term Medical: Temporary coverage for an individual for a short period of time, usually from 30 days to six months.

Small Employer Group: Generally means groups with two but no more than 50 eligible employees. The definition may vary among states.

Special Enrollment Period: A time, triggered by certain specific events, during which you and your dependents must be permitted to sign up for coverage under a group health plan. Employers and group health insurers must make such a period available to employees and their dependents when their family status changes or when their health insurance status changes. Special enrollment periods must last at least 30 days. Enrollment in a health plan during a special enrollment period is not considered late enrollment.

State Mandated Benefits: When a state passes laws requiring that health insurance plans include specific benefits.

Stop-loss: The dollar amount of claims filed for eligible expenses at which point you've paid 100 percent of your out-of-pocket and the insurance begins to pay at 100%. Stop-loss is reached when an insured individual has paid the deductible and reached the out-of-pocket maximum amount of co-insurance.

T

Triple-Option: Insurance plans that offer three options from which an individual may choose. Usually, the three options are: traditional indemnity, an HMO, and a PPO.

U

Underwriter: The company that assumes responsibility for the risk, issues insurance policies and receives premiums.

Usual, Customary and Reasonable (UCR) or Covered Expenses: An amount customarily charged for or covered for similar services and supplies which are medically necessary, recommended by a doctor, or required for treatment.

V

Viatical Settlement: If you have a life insurance policy, you may be able to sell it to pay for care that is not covered under other insurance policies that you may have. Viaticals, also known as life settlements, are reserved for people have experienced a significant decline in health. The term viatical comes from the Latin word, viaticum, which means "provisions for a journey." Essentially, the cash could be used to help pay for the provisions (medical care) for an individual's end-of-life journey. Many people use the money to pay for medical care that isn't covered under their health insurance and for out-of-pocket expenses.

W

Waiting Period: The time you may be required to work for an employer before you are eligible for health benefits. Not all employers require waiting periods. Waiting periods do not count as gaps in health insurance for purposes of determining whether coverage is continuous. If your employer requires a waiting period, your pre-existing condition exclusion period begins on the first day of the waiting period.

Sample Letter
Reasonable Accommodation under the Americans with Disabilities Act [ADA]

Background:

ADA does NOT require that a request for an accommodation be in writing, and does NOT require that the words "reasonable accommodation" be used. A request for an accommodation is valid whether it is verbal or written, and you do not have to use any special wording. If you do choose to write a letter, however, you will have a record of what you asked for and when. You may also wish to use the words "reasonable accommodation" or even "reasonable accommodation under Title I of the Americans with Disabilities Act" to be very clear about the reason for the request. You may find that your employer has already developed a process for requesting an on-the-job accommodation, and may have a form for you to complete. If not, you may wish to write a letter requesting accommodation. The Job Accommodation Network (1-800-526-7234 or www.jan.wvu.edu) can be very helpful in determining workable options if the need is not obvious.

SAMPLE LETTER
Reasonable Accommodation under the Americans with Disabilities Act [ADA]

Letter Contents:

Date
Attention: Human Resource Manager
Your Employer's Name and Address
Re: Your Name and Job Title

Dear (name):

(Content to consider in the body of your letter)

- Identify yourself as a person with a disability.

- State that you are requesting accommodation under Title I of the Americans with Disabilities Act.

- Identify the specific job tasks that you're having problems with.

- List your accommodation ideas.

- Request your employer's accommodation ideas. (For example, "Please let me know what other accommodation ideas you might have.")

- Ask that your employer respond to your request in a reasonable amount of time (and ask for the response in writing, if you choose), or ask, "When may we meet to discuss this issue?"

SAMPLE LETTER
Reasonable Accommodation under the Americans with Disabilities Act [ADA]

- Refer to medical documentation that you have attached to the letter, or state that you will provide documentation upon request.

- Consider sending copies of the letter to appropriate parties (e.g. managers, human resource personnel), particularly if prior requests have not been acknowledged.

Sincerely,

(your signature)

Your printed name and contact information

CC List other people who are also receiving copies of this request letter

Sample Letter
Family Medical Leave Act Request

Background:

If you want to take FMLA leave, the law requires that you provide the following information to your employer:

- you provide 30-day advance notice of the need to take FMLA leave when the need is foreseeable (such as leave for a new child, or for a planned medical treatment for yourself or a family member); or

- you provide notice "as soon as practicable" when the need to take FMLA leave is not foreseeable. "As soon as practicable" generally means at least verbal notice to the employer *within one or two business days* of learning of the need to take FMLA leave;

The law also requires that:

- you provide sufficient information for the employer to understand that you need leave for FMLA-qualifying reasons. In other words, you do not need to mention FMLA when requesting leave, but must only explain why the leave is needed; and

- where the employer was not made aware that an employee was absent for FMLA reasons and the employee wants the leave counted as FMLA leave, the employee should give timely notice (generally *within two business days* of returning to work) that leave was taken for an FMLA-qualifying reason.

Employers may also require employees to provide medical certification supporting the need for leave due to a serious health condition that is affecting the employee or an immediate family member. Employers can also require second or third medical opinions, at the employer's expense, and periodic recertification that the need for leave (the serious health condition) still exists. You may also be asked during FMLA leave to provide periodic reports regarding your status and intent to return to work.

Sample Letter
Family Medical Leave Act Request

Letter Contents:

Date
Attention: Human Resource Manager
Your Employer's Name and Address
Re: Your Name and Job Title

Dear (name)

(Content to consider in the body of your letter)

- Give enough information to your company explaining why you are requesting this leave such as for birth or adoption, for your own serious health condition, or for the serious health condition of your child, spouse, or parent. In this instance you are requesting leave to treat your condition of breast cancer.

- In your request for leave, you do not have to give detailed personal information. Your employer, however, may request more information through a medical certification form that they may ask you to fill out.

- Mention in your letter that you want to take this leave under the Family Medical Leave Act (FMLA), so that your employer can not say that it did not know you were requesting FMLA leave.

SAMPLE LETTER
Family Medical Leave Act Request

• Identify the date you want the leave to begin and project the date that you will believe it will end. If you do not provide the proper notice, then your employer may deny leave, delay the start of leave, or terminate you for taking leave without authorization. You must comply with notice and certification requirements under FMLA in order to take advantage of your right.

Sincerely,

Your Name and Signature

Your Contact information

cc (List other people who will receive copies of this letter such as your immediate supervisor.)

Reprint permission granted from Workplace Fairness (www.workplacefairness.org)

Sample Medical
Necessary Appeal Letter

Background:

If you and your provider (most likely a physician) have sent a letter asking for your insurance company to cover a treatment or procedure for you and the company denied your request, then approach the provider who made this request on your behalf and ask them to send the following type of letter.

Letter Contents:

Date
Attention: Medical Director
Your Insurance Company
Address
RE: Your Name
Your Policy Number
Proposed Treatment:

Dear Medical Director,

I recently learned as a result of your denial letter of *(date and any case numbers assigned to the denial)* requesting preauthorization of the above referenced treatment that you do not consider the care I proposed for *(your name)* as medically necessary. I would like to better understand the rationale for your denial, thus please provide the following information:

SAMPLE MEDICAL
Necessary Appeal Letter

· Name and credentials of the medical professional who reviewed the treatment records.

· A listing of the specific records that you reviewed regarding this case.

· Copies of any expert medical opinions you secured regarding this treatment and how it relates to this case.

I would like to know what alternative treatment your company proposes for my patient, *(your name)* with the appropriate medical back-up that supports this decision. Your immediate response is requested and appreciated.

Sincerely,

Your Provider's Name

Note: If your physician provider will not send this letter, then you may send it yourself making the appropriate changes. Enclose a copy of the denial letter.

INDEX